SYPHILIS

a synopsis

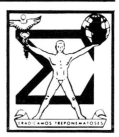

ERADICAMOS TREPONEMATOSES

U.S. DEPARTMENT OF
HEALTH, EDUCATION, AND WELFARE
Public Health Service

Bureau of Disease Prevention and Environmental Control
National Communicable Disease Center • Venereal Disease Program
Atlanta, Georgia   30333

The Public Health Service gratefully acknowledges the assistance of Drs. Martin M. Abbrecht, Terrence E. Billings, Bobby C. Brown, Carl J. Cohen, Eugene J. Gillespie, Charles L. Heaton, James B. Lucas, Dee M. Rasmussen, Kirk D. Wuepper, and Mr. Kenneth P. Latimer in the preparation of this manuscript. Credit is also due Drs. Lewis M. Drusin, C. Wendell Freeman, E. Randolph Wilkerson, Jr., and Phillip M. Utley for many of the photographs which appear herein.

Special appreciation is extended to Dr. Herman Beerman and Dr. Harry Pariser for their painstaking review of the manuscript.

Public Health Service Publication No. 1660
January 1968

U.S. Government Printing Office, Washington, D.C.: 1967

For sale by the Superintendent of Documents, U.S. Government Printing Office
Washington, D.C., 20402 — Price $ 2.00

FOREWORD

The purpose of this book is to bring to its readers a concise presentation of current knowledge and recent developments in the diagnosis and treatment of syphilis. It is hoped that the text supplemented by visual aids will be instructive — particularly to practicing physicians and to students of medicine in their study of syphilis.

At this point in time, reported cases of infectious syphilis have leveled off, and in fact have shown a slight decline. During this transition period and subsequent years, we must be particularly vigilant to avoid the serious mistake made in the 1950's when significant decreases in reported syphilis lead to a tragic de-emphasis of the control of this disease —only to be followed by its recrudescence.

Although the search for a vaccine has not been successful to date, it is fortunate that penicillin is still efficacious in the treatment of this infection. However, past experience has taught us that penicillin alone is not enough. Syphilis control depends on a combination of factors including a high index of suspicion, clinical acumen, laboratory tests, diagnosis, treatment, case reporting, and epidemiology. In addition to interviewing patients for sexual contacts and follow-up by trained health department personnel, the epidemiologic (preventive) treatment of sexual contacts exposed to infectious syphilis, even though negative on initial examination, is essential to successful control.

With teamwork between private physicians and health officers, a lasting victory over the treponeme of syphilis, which has plagued human beings for so long a time, is inevitable.

William J. Brown

WILLIAM J. BROWN, M.D.
Chief, Venereal Disease Program
National Communicable Disease Center

CONTENTS

List of Illustrations

Chapter II.—Pathophysiology of Syphilis

Chapter IV.—Primary Syphilis

Chapter V.—Secondary Syphilis

Chapter VI.—Epidemiology of Syphilis

Chapter VII.—Late Syphilis

Chapter VIII.—Congenital Syphilis

Chapter I.—HE WHO KNOWS SYPHILIS

"HE WHO KNOWS SYPHILIS, KNOWS MEDICINE."
Sir William Osler

This introductory chapter does not purport to be a compre-
hensive history of syphilis, for few diseases, if any, have a
more detailed and well chronicled history. It is hoped, however, that through this brief historical outline the reader will
gain an appropriate appreciation of the continuing menace
and challenge that syphilis still poses to mankind and to
medical science.

For nearly half a millennium scholars and medical his-
torians have debated the mysterious origin of syphilis. Thus
an academic dispute has evolved over whether syphilis
originated in the New World (Columbian Theory) or had
been present in the Old World from time immemorial
(Pre-Columbian Theory).

The Columbian school believes that syphilitic infection
was endemic in Hispaniola (Haiti) and was subsequently
contracted and carried to Europe by Columbus' crew when
they returned to Spain following his second voyage. Columbus departed Seville in August 1492, and following his visit
to Hispaniola returned to Palos Bay on March 15, 1493.
In the company of six sailors and six Indians he then travel-
ed from Palos to Barcelona by way of Seville. This group
of travelers plus the majority of sailors who remained at
Palos are believed to be the nidus for the syphilization of
Europe.

In late 1494, King Charles VIII of France besieged Naples. In his army were Spanish mercenaries as well as soldiers of fortune from nearly every country in Europe. (Syphilis was said to be already present among the Neapolitans.) Shortly after the fall of the city, syphilis became widespread throughout the army and Italy. When this new disease first appeared in Charles' army, those French troops showing evidence of syphilis were returned to their homeland and without doubt served to spread the infection en route.

Scholars adhering to the Pre-Columbian Theory affirm just as vehemently that syphilis had been present in Europe prior to the voyage of Columbus but was either unrecognized, confused with other diseases (probably leprosy), or was present in a much milder form. Hudson and others feel that the infection probably originated in Central Africa as a yaws-like illness, and was eventually introduced into Europe by travelers and traders. In Europe syphilis gradually acquired a venereal mode of transmission and many of the clinical characteristics of the present-day disease.

Whatever its origin, there can be no question that a great pandemic of syphilis suddenly appeared in all parts of Europe and that by 1497 the disease had appeared even in as remote an area as Scotland. At this time syphilis was apparently a very acute disease, frequently fatal in the secondary stage. It was almost immediately recognized as being a new and previously unknown condition, and as early as 1500 many physicians throughout Europe were reporting and describing its symptoms. Fortunately, the extremely acute, severe form of syphilis apparently became rather quickly attenuated to the more chronic form of today.

It is obvious that neither theory of the origin of syphilis is entirely satisfactory. Not only is it difficult to conceive how the disease could spread so rapidly from a single port of entry, but it is equally difficult to accept the conclusion

2

that a previously endemic disease could so suddenly become epidemic and could develop previously unknown characteristics with an entirely new degree of severity.

In the closing years of the 15th century descriptions of the disease began to appear in the literature of the day. The first mention of the new disease is found in an edict issued by the Diet of Worms on October 7, 1495. It was referred to as *bösen blattern* (the evil pox). As early as 1497 mercury was being advocated by at least two physicians, Johannes Widmann and Corradino Gilino, and in 1498 the first major book on syphilis was written by Francisco Lopez de Villalobos. He recognized the venereal mode of transmission and described the skin manifestations and later complications of syphilis. He also deduced the idea of treatment with mercury from a study of the old Arabic literature.

In 1514 Juan de Vigo described with amazing clinical accuracy the stages of the disease, including discussions and descriptions of gummatous syphilis. However, the late lesions of cardiovascular and central nervous system syphilis were not associated with the disease during this early period. It was in 1532 that Niccolo Massa, an Italian physician, described certain of the neurological effects of syphilis. About 200 years later, in 1728, Giovanni Maria Lancisi (1654-1720) in a posthumously published text on aneurysms clearly implicated syphilis as a frequent cause of cardiovascular disease.

At the outset syphilis was known by a variety of names, some of which were derived from the designation of a particular political enemy at a particular point in time. Thus, in France syphilis was known as *"le mal de Naples";* in Naples, "the French disease"; and in England, as "the Spanish disease." Other names—*bösen blattern, Las Bubas, la gross verole* or "the Great Pox"—were used to describe syphilis in medical literature of the day.

In 1530 an Italian pathologist, Hieronymus Fracas-

3

torius, wrote a poem entitled *"Syphilis Sive Morbus Gallicus,"* which described the plight of a mythical shepherd lad named Syphilus afflicted with the French disease as punishment for cursing the gods. The poem recognized the venereal nature of the infection and was a compendium of knowledge of the time regarding the disease.

While he did not publish his findings until 1539, Rodrigo Ruy de Isla mentions that he first recognized the malady among the sailors of Columbus' crew and attributed its origin to the Island of Espanola. It is also noteworthy that he observed the beneficial effects of fever on the course of the disease.

The first English writer to broach the subject of syphilis was William Clowes who in 1579 published a treatise on venereal disease. His descriptions indicate that the course of syphilis was much milder at that time. Clowes still referred to the disease as the *Morbus Neapolitanus.* It was the English surgeon Thomas Gale who in 1563 actually introduced the word *syphilis* into the English language.

The occurrence of syphilis in the newborn was suspected in even the earliest accounts of the disease and is mentioned by both Lopez and Fracastorius. However, contemporary writers of that age felt that the infection was contracted through infected milk or at the time of parturition. The employment of wet nurses by families of social prominence was common practice and without doubt many of these women were infected. Paracelsus seems to have been the first to assert that syphilis must have been acquired *in utero.* He and others for several centuries to come felt that the father was capable of directly infecting the developing ovum, since it was obvious that many mothers appeared to be uninfected. This concept was not abandoned until the introduction of serologic tests in the 20th century. However, both Trousseau in 1846 and Cullerier in 1854 felt that the mother must have acquired the infection before transmission to a child was possible. As early as 1565

4

Simon de Vallambert, a French pediatrician, devoted an entire chapter in one of his works to syphilis in children. The Irish surgeon Abraham Colles (1773-1843) observed that infected infants could not produce breast ulcerations when suckled by their mother. This has since become known as Colles' law and certainly suggests that Colles suspected that the mother's resistance to syphilis probably was due to her preceding infection.

In France, P. Diday concerned himself primarily with congenital syphilis and in 1854 published a nearly complete account of infantile signs and symptoms. He did not recognize that the infection could be latent in children and believed that children who did not display symptoms by six months of age were uninfected.

Sir Jonathan Hutchinson (1828-1913) is probably the best remembered student of congenital syphilis. His studies on the stigmata of late congenital syphilis are classic. He established the fact that interstitial keratitis is almost always due to congenital syphilis. He was the first to describe the most characteristic of the syphilitic dental malformations which bear his name, and he pointed out the frequent association of notched incisors, interstitial keratitis, and eighth nerve deafness—Hutchinson's triad.

The concept of latency in both acquired and congenital syphilis was propounded by Jean Alfred Fournier (1832-1914) who clarified many misconceptions concerning the disease and first taught, in an era when direct proof was lacking, that tabes dorsalis and general paralysis of the insane or paresis were the result of antecedent syphilis. In 1874 Jean-Martin Charcot described the gastric crisis and destructive trophic joint changes associated with tabes dorsalis.

R. Bertin, G. Wegner, and J. Parrott all made important contributions to the knowledge of the bone lesions caused by syphilitic osteochondritis, and in 1886 H. H. Clutton reported the painless symmetrical hydrarthrosis of the knee joints associated with late congenital syphilis. The counterpart of Clutton's joints, occasionally seen in adults with acquired syphilis, was described by Aristide August Verneuil.

There can be little doubt that after syphilis first appeared in Europe the early lesions were frequently confused with other venereal as well as nonvenereal diseases. Mixed or superimposed infections were unquestionably common in periods when personal hygiene left much to be desired. Indeed, mixed infections are by no means rare today. In an extant record written in 1496, the German physician Joseph Grunpeck described mixed as well as multiple syphilitic primary lesions. That other skin conditions should have been confused with syphilis is readily understood. But it is much more difficult to comprehend the confusion of syphilis and gonorrhea which appears to have developed almost immediately upon the recognition of the former disease in the last years of the 15th century.

Descriptions of gonorrhea by Guillaume de Salicet and John of Arderne in the 13th and 14th centuries leave little doubt that this infection was not only prevalent and recognized as venereal in origin, but was also regarded in those times as a separate disease entity. However, by 1530 Paracelsus was teaching that gonorrhea was an initial symptom of syphilis. Controversy eventually developed around the duality concept of these two diseases and debate continued until the self-experimentation of John Hunter in 1767.

Hunter was probably the greatest figure in experimental medicine and biology of his century in addition to being a surgeon of great fame. He obtained pus from a patient with gonorrhea and inoculated himself. It was most unfortunate that the inoculum was contaminated with the causative organism of syphilis as well, and both syphilis and gonorrhea developed in typical fashion. Despite mercurial inunctions for the cutaneous syphilids, he developed classic

6

syphilitic heart disease, which ultimately caused his death in 1793. While he was not the first to describe its characteristics, his name is associated with the true or hard chancre of syphilis. He failed in other experiments to transmit the disease to volunteers, in all probability because they had been previously infected and were immune. When Hunter's book entitled *Treatise on the Venereal Diseases* was published in 1787 his reputation was such that the entire subject of concurrent infection was obtunded for a half century despite the publication in 1793 of a *Treatise on Gonorrhea Virulenta and Lues Venerea,* by Benjamin Bell, which clearly differentiated the two diseases. Bell was himself a famous Scottish surgeon and demonstrated the distinctness of the two conditions by experimentation on himself and medical students.

The credit for finally changing medical thought and delineating syphilis and gonorrhea belongs to Philippe Ricord, a Frenchman, although American by birth. He was an investigator of the first rank but, unlike Hunter, devoted his research primarily to the venereal diseases. Ricord's report in 1838, based on over 2,500 human inoculations, demonstrated conclusively that syphilis and gonorrhea were distinct diseases. He very carefully characterized the stages of syphilis and provided the terms still used for the classification of the disease, i.e., primary, secondary, and tertiary. He realized, as Hunter had not, that reinfection was a rarity, and by reintroducing the vaginal speculum to clinical medicine he demonstrated vaginal and cervical lesions. Ricord felt, as had his predecessors, that mercury was the therapeutic agent of choice. However, when William Wallace, an Irish physician, in 1836 introduced potassium iodide as a new form of therapy for syphilis, Ricord quickly realized its value and succeeded in popularizing its use in France. Wallace, who was a somewhat quarrelsome individualist, also made a second important contribution by investigating and proving by inoculation the contagiousness of secondary lesions which were formerly thought to be incapable of transmitting the disease.

For centuries no specific etiology had been assigned to syphilis. Many of the earliest writers who were also astrologers blamed the disease upon a malignant alignment of the stars and planets. In a later age, diseases, including syphilis, were ascribed to a lack of balance among the humors of the body. With the pioneering work of Pasteur, Koch, Löeffler and others, the world entered the bacteriological era, and a hysterical search to discover the cause of syphilis began. Numerous bacteria were reported as being causal, but scientists were unable to confirm or repeat the critical experiments.

The five-year period 1905-10 heralded a trinity of discoveries that ushered in the modern age of syphilis management; the discovery of T. pallidum, the advent of serologic tests for syphilis and the development of arsphenamine therapy.

Elie Metchnikoff and Emile Roux successfully transmitted the infection to monkeys in 1903 and made possible the experimental study of syphilis. In 1905 Albert Neisser, who had previously discovered the gonococcus, extended the work of Metchnikoff and Roux by establishing a primate colony in Batavia, Java, where he studied the problem of immunity in syphilis, and its experimental therapy and pathology. However, it remained for Fritz Schaudinn and Erich Hoffmann, working together at the Reichsgesundheitsamt in Berlin, to discover the spiral organism in serum from a lesion of secondary syphilis. In 1905 they reported that syphilis was caused by a spirochete which they named *Spirochaeta pallida*. This work was quickly confirmed when Karl Landsteiner introduced the darkfield method for the detection of the organism in 1906. In that same year, Karl Reuter, a German physician, found *Treponema pallidum* in the wall of a syphilitic aorta, and in 1913 Hideyo Noguchi was able to transmit syphilis to rabbits by the inoculation of brain tissue from paretics. This established beyond all doubt that paresis was a late manifestation of syphilis.

By 1906 the principles of the complement fixation test, demonstrated by Jules Bordet and Octave Gengou, awaited application. August von Wassermann and his co-workers, Albert Neisser and Carl Bruck, quickly applied this test method to the study of serum of syphilitic patients. They prepared their antigen from the liver of a stillborn congenital syphilitic infant. The following year Marie and Levaditi demonstrated that saline extracts on nonsyphilitic organs could serve equally well for the purpose of obtaining antigens. While Wassermann's test was a great advance, allowing the detection and treatment of millions of previously undiagnosed syphilitics, a constant search for more sensitive and specific tests continues to this day. Since the time of Wassermann's work over 200 different serologic procedures for syphilis diagnosis have been described. Each has generally been named for its author serologist.

Once animal experimentation with syphilis had been successfully established and the organism identified, a systematic approach to therapy could begin. Dr. Paul Ehrlich, the famous physician-chemist, turned his attention to this problem in 1909, the year after he was awarded the Nobel Prize for basic work in immunology.

Mercury, as previously mentioned, came into use in the treatment of syphilis about 1497. This drug had many vicissitudes of fortune during its long use. It was at various times applauded as the remedy *par excellence* and at other times condemned as a noxious poison. The problem lay with the huge doses which were frequently administered and which led to mercurialism or mercury poisoning. Symptoms of mercury poisoning were so common that they were considered as part of the tertiary stage of syphilis by many early syphilologists. So bad was the reputation of mercury during the period from 1580 to 1655 that every teacher in the University of Heidelberg was required to take an oath that he would never use any form of the drug. Nevertheless, mercury continued to command the attention of physicians and had its advocates, in mixed therapy, until the advent of penicillin. With the exception of potassium iodide, mercury was the only truly efficacious therapy known until Ehrlich introduced arsphenamine (Salvarsan, or 606) into clinical practice in 1910.

In the early days of the 20th century sleeping sickness was a major problem confronting the German colonization of Africa. To combat this problem Ehrlich had been investigating numerous compounds for effectiveness against experimental trypanosomiasis as early as 1902. Atoxyl, a compound originally synthesized by Bechamp in 1863 first stimulated Ehrlich's interest in the organic arsenical compounds. Atoxyl had been shown to be spirocheticidal in chicken spirillosis by Uhlenhuth and was eventually tried in human syphilis. While the results were encouraging it was found that Atoxyl produced a high incidence of optic atrophy. Nonetheless, these experiments encouraged Ehrlich to synthesize a long list of related arsenic derivatives. All of these new compounds were immediately tested in animals for spirocheticidal activity and toxic effects. By 1907 Ehrlich had reached the 606th preparation in the series. While this compound (Arsphenamine, or Salvarsan) was patented, it was put aside after an assistant reported that it had not proved effective in animal experiments.

Fully two years later, in 1909, Professor Kitasato of Tokyo sent a pupil, Dr. Sahachiro Hata, to study with Ehrlich. Hata was particularly skilled in experimental syphilis, and beginning with compound number 418 which had shown some promise, he repeated the previous assistant's experiments. Hata demonstrated that compound 606 was highly efficacious and in September of that same year clinical trials under Professor Konrad Alt were begun. Arsphenamine or "606" was quickly shown to be far superior to mercury and soon became the drug of choice in syphilis therapy. Although the drug demonstrated true and rapid spirocheticidal activity, clinical cure required repeated injections over a period of one and one-half years. Ehrlich was not content with "606" and continued his investigations until his death in 1915. Although product "914" or Neosalvarsan was more soluble in water and neutral in reaction, neither it nor a host of other arsenic derivatives were ever proven to be more effective than "606".

Felix Balzer in 1889 suggested the use of bismuth compounds based on animal experiments. However, favorable results were not reported in human syphilis until the work of Sazerac and Levaditi who in 1922 described their findings based on the treatment of 200 cases in all stages of the disease. While not as active as arsenicals, bismuth preparations proved to be far less toxic. Soon after the advent of bismuth into syphilotherapy, the alternate use of arsenicals and bismuth compounds became the popular mode of treatment of syphilis. By the time pencillin became available, the number of commercially available bismuth preparations had proliferated into the hundreds.

While the heavy metals (mercurials, bismuth preparations, and arsenicals) were effective and usually curative in the earlier stages of syphilis, some stages of late syphilis, particularly dementia paralytica or paresis, proved refractory to all forms of therapy. It had been known for many years that fevers often had a favorable influence on the course of psychotic patients. As mentioned previously, this phenomenon had been observed by Ruy de Isla centuries before. However, the credit for introducing and developing fever therapy belongs to Julius von Wagner-Jauregg, a Viennese psychiatrist. Wagner-Jauregg studied many forms of artificial fever production and in 1917 began his first classical studies on the effect of malarial inoculation. A successful malarial treatment produced temperatures of 103

11

to 106 degrees F. lasting from 6 to 12 hours. Usually the patient was permitted to have 10-12 paroxysms before termination of treatment with quinine. *Plasmodium vivax* was usually the malarial parasite chosen because of its sensitivity to quinine. Malarial therapy was no panacea for the paretic and in unselected cases only 20-30 percent of patients obtained complete lasting remissions. Nonetheless, fever therapy represented an important advance in the management of these heretofore hopeless patients. In 1927 Wagner-Jauregg received the Nobel Prize in Medicine for his achievement. Later the Kettering electronic cabinet became widely used in the United States and produced results nearly equaling those of malaria therapy.

In all probability the greatest single therapeutic advance in the history of infectious disease was Sir Alexander Fleming's discovery of penicillin from the fungus *Penicillium notatum*. In 1943, John Friend Mahoney reported the remarkable results obtained with penicillin in the treatment of four patients with primary syphilis. The healing of lesions was little short of miraculous, and as quickly as supplies of penicillin became available other workers confirmed Mahoney's results. Within a short period of time penicillin had completely supplanted all other forms of therapy in the treatment of syphilis in any stage of the disease. While other drugs have replaced it in the treatment of many nonspirochetal diseases, penicillin remains the drug of choice 25 years after its introduction by Mahoney.

The problem of individual prophylaxis and suggested measures to be taken following exposure are included as a part of nearly every early treatise on syphilis. Later writers, particularly during the latter half of the 19th century, frequently concerned themselves with the question of adequate treatment and the advisability of marriage following infection. The actual concept of control in a broad public health sense was largely ignored. To be sure, primitive control measures and statutes directing the incarceration and quarantine of persons (usually prostitutes) thought to be infectious have existed for centuries.

Control of syphilis could not become a reality until the tools to implement the concept were at hand. The dramatic identification of *T. pallidum* by Schaudinn and Hoffmann in 1905, the introduction of the Wassermann reaction the following year, and the development of "606" by Ehrlich in 1909-10 provided the knowledge from which a national control program could be devised. The impetus required for the synthesis of national programs can probably be traced to the problems created by the outbreak of World War I. It was quickly discovered when the United States entered the War that venereal disease constituted a major cause of rejection for the armed services. While all evidence indicates that the number of persons already infected with syphilis was immense (for example, approximately one American in ten), syphilis undoubtedly became even more prevalent during the war years.

In 1918 Congress passed the Chamberlain-Kahn Act which created the Venereal Disease Division of the U.S. Public Health Service. The war ended before a lasting impact on venereal disease could be achieved and the funds subsequently allotted ·to the Venereal Disease Division quickly dwindled. By the mid 1930's only a meager and ineffective national program existed, despite the fact that the number of reported cases was significantly higher than in the preceding decade.

A revitalization of the national program and a public awakening to the scope of the problem occurred with the appointment of Dr. Thomas Parran as Surgeon General in 1936. Dr. Parran had earlier been in charge of the Venereal Disease Division of the Public Health Service, and he immediately supported a broadly based publicity campaign calling attention to the ravages and costs of uncontrolled syphilis. For the first time the facts became accessible to the people through the media of newspapers, magazines, and radio. Dr. Parran finally succeeded in making syphilis an acceptable word in society. In December 1936 a National Venereal Disease Conference was held in Washington and attended by more than a thousand of the nation's most prominent leaders in medicine, business, and civic affairs. This conference pointed out the need for a long-range control program and the importance of community demonstrations to show how effective action, with cooperation of the physician, public health worker, and citizenry, could be carried out. Public interest continued and demonstration projects were started through grants-in-aid to individual states, a pattern that has been followed since that time.

As a result of the national attention focused on the problem, Congress in 1938 unanimously passed the National Venereal Disease Control Act, which had been sponsored in the Senate by Robert M. LaFollette and in the House by Alfred L. Bulwinkle. This peace-time act implied a long-term attack on syphilis and provided for the first time since World War I ample appropriations for the task.

If World War I had served as a stimulus for the formation of national venereal disease control effort, the advent of the Second World War demonstrated its absolute necessity. Of the 12 million men called to service over 170,000 required treatment for syphilis before being placed on active duty. To quickly cure infected men for the draft and to concomitantly treat the civilian population without hindering the war effort required new approaches. Special therapy facilities, known as rapid treatment centers, were established throughout the country by the Lanham Act passed in 1943. These centers provided intensive, often continuous drip therapy with arsenical preparations, and a schedule of full treatment could be accomplished in from only 5-10 days as compared to the usual 70-week course given in outpatient clinics. Controls were also established to treat infected men prior to their discharge to civilian life. Thus

14

between November 1944 and October 1946 over 50,000 men were treated before release.

Shortly after the close of World War II, 63 rapid treatment centers had been established and were annually treating 185,000 persons with all stages of syphilis. Many patients were brought to the rapid treatment centers as a result of mass serologic testing. Despite this, in 1947 over 106,000 cases of infectious syphilis were reported.

The idea of case prevention through spread control began in the rapid treatment centers and has slowly evolved into the modern day concepts of patient interviewing and contact tracing.

With the widespread availability of penicillin, and particularly its longer acting forms, inpatient care was no longer necessary and the rapid treatment centers were closed. During this same period of the late 1940's and early 1950's a dramatic drop in national syphilis morbidity was recorded. The cause for this drop in incidence remains an enigma, but in all probability the nonspecific use of penicillin for nearly every condition, which was so prevalent in those years, resulted in the coincidental cure of many patients. Penicillin, indeed, appeared to be a panacea and many felt during the early 1950's that syphilis would shortly disappear. However, this was not to be the case. After a low of approximately 6,500 cases annually for the period 1955-57, the incidence of infectious syphilis once again began to climb and by 1963 exceeded 22,000.

To cope with the tide of new cases which were increasing at a rate of 50 percent per year, Surgeon General Luther Terry appointed a Task Force in 1961 to review the syphilis problem and to recommend a course of action. Late in that year the Task Force set forth a number of basic steps, which if fully implemented would result in the eradication of syphilis as a public health hazard in the United States within the following decade.

Presently, the rising incidence of infectious syphilis has

been stemmed. The next few years will tell whether this disease can be eradicated in the United States. This high goal will be a hopeless one unless supported by every physician whose pledge of cooperation is unequivocally needed to achieve this end. Physicians must not only be able to diagnose and treat syphilis, but to reach this goal they must report every case to local health authorities and grant permission for their patients to be interviewed by competent health department personnel. It is also a prerequisite for eradication that all sexual contacts to infectious syphilis found not to be infected on initial examination be given prophylactic treatment.

Bibliography

1. ANDERSON, ODIN W.: Syphilis and Society—Problems of Control in the United States, 1912-64. Center for Health Administration Studies, Health Information Foundation, Research Series 22. Chicago, University of Chicago Press, 1965.

2. DENNIE, C. C.: A History of Syphilis. Springfield, Illinois, Charles C. Thomas, 1962.

3. GOODMAN, H.: Notable Contributors to the Knowledge of Syphilis. New York, Froben Press, 1943.

4. HUDSON, E. H.: Treponematosis and anthropology. Ann. Int. Med., 58:1037-1048, 1963.

5. The Eradication of Syphilis: A Task Force Report to the Surgeon General, Public Health Service, on Syphilis Control in the United States. PHS Publ. 918. Washington, D.C., U.S. Government Printing Office, 1962.

Chapter II.—PATHOPHYSIOLOGY
OF SYPHILIS

Biology of Treponema Pallidum

The causative organism of syphilis is a member of the order *Spirochaetales* and the family *Treponemataceae*. The many members of the order *Spirochaetales* are widely distributed in nature with the overwhelming majority being free-living or saprophytic. Numerous species have been described in soil, water and in the alimentary tracts of insects and amphibians. The spirochetes are generally defined as actively motile organisms whose motion is produced not by flagella but by means of a corkscrew rotation.

The family *Treponemataceae* contains three genera: The *Borrelia*, the *Treponema,* and the *Leptospira.* Members of all three genera are parasitic or pathogenic for man, other mammals, and/or birds. The genus *Treponema* contains four principal species of pathogenic organisms: *T. pallidum,* the organism responsible for human syphilis; *T. pertenue* and *T. carateum,* the etiologic agents of yaws and pinta, respectively; and *T. cuniculi,* which is responsible for rabbit syphilis.

Although these organisms are all morphologically and serologically identical, they can be distinguished antigenically from the nonpathogenic cultivatable strains of *Treponema* such as *T. microdentium.* The evolution of the pathogenic treponemes is a matter of speculation. Most authors believe that they developed from free-living, nonpathogenic forms, and later adapted to their human or

17

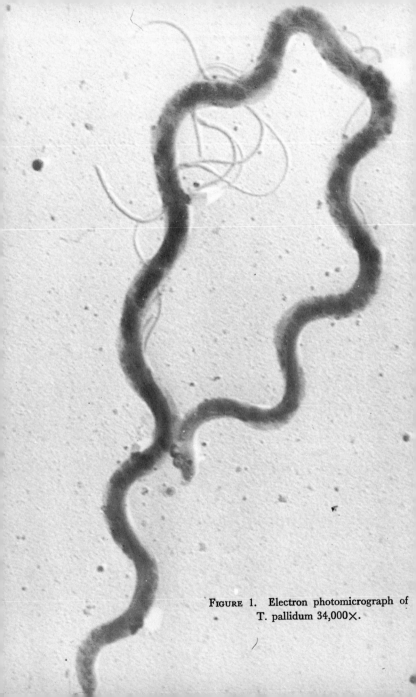

FIGURE 1. Electron photomicrograph of T. pallidum 34,000×.

animal hosts. Although it is suggested that all of the pathogenic *Treponema* were derived from a single source, speculations differ as to how far back in the evolutionary scale the differentiation between them occurred. Many authors think that all *Treponema* pathogenic to humans are the same organisms modified only by various factors in the environment and host.

Treponema pallidum is a thin, delicate organism with tapering ends. It varies from about 6 to 15 microns in length (approximately the diameter of a normal red blood cell), and is of a uniform cylindrical thickness of approximately 0.25 micron. The organisms usually present between 6 and 14 spirals (Figure 1). The ends are pointed with finely spiral terminal filaments, believed by some authorities to be remnants of fission. While *Treponema pallidum* usually conforms to this general morphology it must be emphasized that a more important criterion for its differentiation is its motility as described under "Darkfield Examination," page 43. Despite the conformance of this organism to both morphological and mobility criteria, it still may be impossible to differentiate it from nonpathologenic saprophytic forms and other pathogenic treponemes. In the final analysis the entire spectrum of information, including clinical picture, site of origin of the organism, as well as the morphology and the motility, is necessary to arrive at a definitive decision.

Investigation of *Treponema pallidum* with the electron microscope shows it to resemble a two-strand electric flex with a thin bundle of fibrils wound around a wide central core. In addition, the entire organism is surrounded by a delicate sheath known as the **periplast** or **periblast**. The number of fibrils usually number between 3 and 6. Biochemically the organism is composed of a protein, a polysaccharide, and two different lipids. The difficulty of obtaining sufficiently purified organisms, however, hampers exact chemical definition.

19

Despite claims to the contrary, *Treponema pallidum* has not been maintained outside the human or animal hosts. There are a number of avirulent strains designated as *Treponema pallidum* which have been maintained in artificial media for many years. These organisms were supposedly derived from syphilitic lesions and initially were thought to be virulent, but this virulence was subsequently lost. These include the Reiter, the Noguchi, the Nichols nonpathogenic, and a number of Kazan strains. Most authors today, however, believe that the cultured strains were either picked up accidentally as saprophytic treponemes in the original cultures or that they have become remote variants of *Treponema pallidum* during their many generations of *in vitro* culture. Attempts to culture *Treponema pallidum* in tissue culture or in embryonating eggs have also met with failure. The organism has, however, been maintained for periods up to 22 days in specially designed maintenance media containing thioglycolate. These organisms are observed to be actively motile over a long period of time. However, this apparent continuation of life and active motility is not synonymous with maintenance of virulence.

The usual method of division of *Treponema pallidum* is thought to be binary transverse fission, although some authorities claim that longitudinal division may occur (Figure 2). Generation time for pathogenic *Treponema pallidum* is computed to be approximately 30 to 33 hours. The development of a bud or sporelike form for both cultured and virulent strains has been reported and proposed as a characteristic phase of the life cycle of these organisms. These buds develop along the lateral border of the organism and form cysts from which new treponemes may theoretically emerge. However, it has been shown that these forms are usually encountered under adverse environmental conditions, for example, osmotic shock, heat, or excessive aeration, and thus may not be reproductive forms.

20

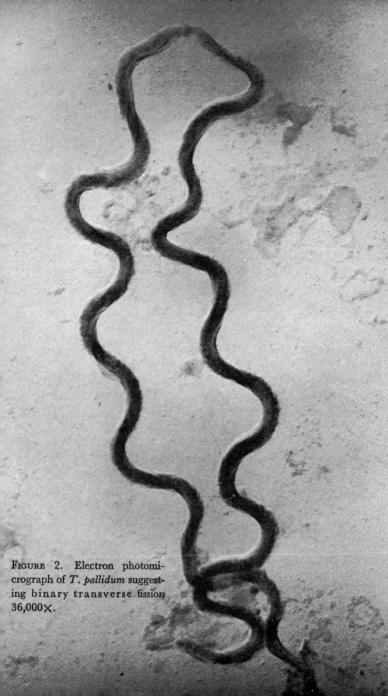

FIGURE 2. Electron photomicrograph of *T. pallidum* suggesting binary transverse fission 36,000×.

Outside of the host *Treponema pallidum* is extremely susceptible to a variety of physical and chemical agents which rapidly bring about its destruction. Heat, drying, soap and water, and storage at refrigerator temperature bring about the destruction of this organism. Despite this frailty of the organism, the morphology, motility, and virulence of *Treponema pallidum* have been preserved for many years by freezing at minus 78° C. and storing at this temperature.

Although a number of mammalian species are readily infected by *Treponema pallidum,* the most widely used experimental animal host is the rabbit in which a whole spectrum of disease can be produced, depending on the method of inoculation. The minimal infective dose for this animal is one treponeme (pathogenic Nichols strain) inoculated intratesticularly, or four organisms inoculated intradermally. While early infectious lesions are common late visceral lesions have been only rarely observed.

Natural Course of Syphilis

Syphilis is transmitted through direct contact with an infectious lesion. The spirochetes pass through intact mucous membranes and abraded skin, following which they are carried by the blood stream to every organ of the body. The infection is systemic a few hours after exposure although clinical and serologic evidence of the disease is lacking for a time.

Approximately 3 to 4 weeks (from as few as 10 to as many as 90 days) after the treponeme has gained entrance into a new host, there develops at the portal of entry a primary lesion, the chancre. This persists 1 to 5 weeks and then heals spontaneously. Serologic tests for syphilis are usually nonreactive when the chancre first appears but become reactive during the following 1 to 4 weeks. (See "Serologic Interpretation," page 96.) Approximately half the patients seen during this stage will be seronegative.

22

About 6 weeks later (2 weeks to 6 months), a generalized or localized cutaneous eruption may appear. In some cases this secondary stage of syphilis appears before the chancre has healed. In other cases it may be so minimal and transient that it is never clinically apparent. As with primary syphilis there is spontaneous healing after 2 to 6 weeks. Following healing of the early lesions there ensues a quiescent or latent stage during which there are no clinical signs or symptoms of the disease. About 25 percent of cases will experience at least one cutaneous relapse after the secondary eruption has healed. Serologic tests during this stage are invariably reactive. Hence the stages of secondary syphilis and early latency fluctuate back and forth until certain immunologic changes take place, usually after one year of infection. Serologic tests during these stages are invariably reactive.

The infected individual during the latent stage is recognized as syphilitic only by means of reactive serologic tests. This latent period has been defined arbitrarily in various ways over the years. In the standard definition of latent syphilis as defined by the World Health Organization*, latency is divided into two periods:

Early latent (duration under 4 years).

Late latent (duration 4 years and over).

Studies in syphilis **epidemiology** have recently indicated that only early latent syphilis of under 1 year's duration produces sufficient infectious syphilis to warrant patient interviewing and contact investigation. Because of this finding several state health departments have already changed the definition of early latent syphilis to include only cases of less than 1 year's duration.

---

* *Manual of the International Statistical Classification of Diseases, Injuries, and Causes of Death.* 7th Revision of the International Lists of Diseases and Causes of Death, adopted 1955. Geneva, Switzerland, World Health Organization, 1955.

For statistical purposes, early latent is defined as syphilis of less than four years duration, and late latent is defined as syphilis of more than four years duration. After four years of infection, relapsing infectious lesions similar to those of secondary syphilis are very rare. Latency may last a lifetime or be followed from a few years to 20 years or more by lesions of late syphilis.

Approximately one-third of the people with untreated syphilis will develop late destructive lesions of syphilis (late benign, 17 percent; cardiovascular, 10 percent; central nervous system, 8 percent), and up to 23 percent of the entire group can be expected to die primarily as a result of the disease. Cardiovascular complications account for over 80 percent of the deaths, with the majority of the remaining deaths being due to involvement of the central nervous system.

About two-thirds of the total untreated infected individuals go through life with minimal or no physical inconvenience, although more than one-half of these will remain serologically positive for life. Spontaneous seroreversal is not necessarily synonymous with spontaneous cure, and occasionally patients may have active late manifestation of syphilis but show no reactivity in standard blood tests. Unfortunately, there is no known means of predicting which patients will develop the lesions of late syphilis and which will not.

Treatment changes both the clinical course and serologic pattern of the disease. If the patient is treated adequately before the appearance of the chancre, it is probable that no lesion will appear and that the serologic test for syphilis will remain nonreactive. If treatment occurs during the seronegative primary stage, the serologic test for syphilis usually remains nonreactive and the chancre rapidly heals. On occasion the serologic test may become transiently reactive. Treatment during the seropositive primary stage also results in prompt healing of the chancre and the serologic

24

test usually becomes nonreactive within 12 months. If treatment is delayed until the secondary stage, 90 to 95 percent of patients adequately treated will become serologically nonreactive within 18 months.

Effects of treatment after the secondary stage are variable, but as a rule the sooner the infected person is treated, the more marked and rapid will be the serologic response. The longer the person goes untreated, the longer it will take the serologic test to reach nonreactivity after adequate treatment, if indeed it ever does. Individuals infected 2 years or more before treatment may remain seroreactive for life despite optimum doses of penicillin and clinical cure.

Pathology of Syphilis

As described in the opening paragraph on "Late Syphilis," page 75, the vascular component is the most prominent and persistent feature of this disease. In virtually all stages the arterioles and capillaries show rather characteristic changes of endarteritis and periarteritis. Endarteritis is defined as the swelling and proliferation of the endothelial cells leading to a reduction in the caliber of the vessel lumen, and periarteritis is the proliferation of the adventitial cells and cuffing of the vessel by inflammatory cells consisting of monocytes, plasma cells, and lymphocytes. Furthermore, syphilis may be defined, after tuberculosis, as the classic example of granulomatous inflammation. The gumma, which is characteristic of this basic pathological process, and other pathologic features of syphilis are described as follows:

Primary syphilis: The gross features of primary syphilis are described in Chapter IV, pages 45–46. In the typical primary lesion or chancre the epidermis at the margin of the lesion shows thickening. At the center the epidermis is considerably thinned or may be absent. A lymphocytic and plasmocytic infiltrate is a prominent feature of the dermal changes. There is proliferation of the capillaries and lymphatics. These vessels also show changes of the endarteritic type. The larger vessels exhibit proliferation of all their coats and invasion of their walls by the inflammatory infiltrate. This endarteritic process may be so marked as to result in obliteration of the lumen of some vessels with resulting thrombosis and small areas of necrosis. *Treponema pallidum* can be identified in the lesion by appropriate stains.

Secondary syphilis: The epidermis may vary from no significant change from normal to the rather marked changes seen in the condyloma latum consisting of acanthosis with broadening and elongation of the rete ridges, intracellular and intercellular edema of the rete cells, and migration of neutrophils through the epidermis (Figure 3). The dermal changes, however, are rather consistent for all of the secondary lesions. The superficial and deep vessels show marked endothelial swelling and are surrounded by a pronounced infiltrate consisting of monocytes, plasma cells, and lymphocytes (Figure 4). The number of plasma cells in relation to other inflammatory cells is usually high. *Treponema pallidum* can be identified in the secondary lesions with appropriate stains.

Latent syphilis: By definition no lesions are present in latent syphilis, and the only sign of infection is a reactive serologic test.

Cardiovascular syphilis: Cardiovascular syphilis may be recognized in a number of forms consisting of uncomplicated aortitis; coronary artery ostiastenosis with resulting angina pectoris (Figure 5); aortic regurgitation with its secondary effects on the heart, particularly the left ventricle; and aneurysm. The basic lesion, however, is aortitis with resulting secondary effects on the heart. Involvement of the heart itself is rare, although gummas have been observed in the myocardium (Figure 6). Syphilitic aortitis consists

26

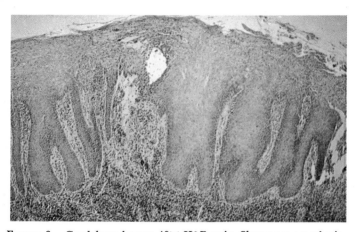

FIGURE 3. Condyloma latum: 40× H&E stain. Shown are acanthosis, broadening and elongation of the rete ridges, intracellular and intercellular edema of the rete cells, and migration of the inflammatory cells through the epidermis. In the dermis there is proliferation of small arterioles showing marked endothelial swelling and a perivascular inflammatory infiltrate.

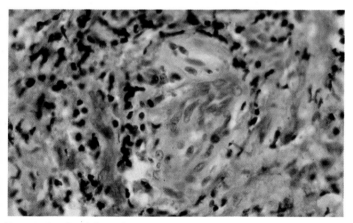

FIGURE 4. Condyloma latum: 400× H&E stain. Marked endothelial proliferation and perivascular inflammatory cuffing characteristically seen in the dermis.

27

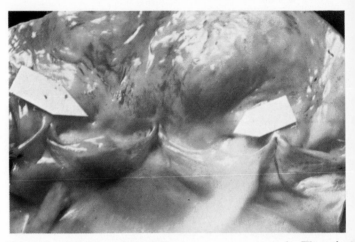

FIGURE 5. Cardiovascular syphilis—coronary artery stenosis: The ostia of both coronary arteries are markedly stenosed. Note "tree-bark" effect in intima of aorta just superior to the valve.

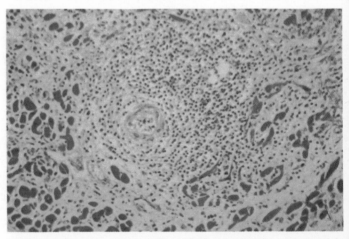

FIGURE 6. Gumma—heart: 950× H&E stain. Microgumma seen in heart with a central zone of necrosis surrounded by large numbers of plasma cells and lymphocytes. Vascular proliferation is present on the periphery.

of necrosis of the media secondary to endarteritis of the vasa vasorum of the wall. Grossly, syphilitic aortitis is characterized by a wrinkled bark-like patchy appearance in a pearly white intima (Figure 7). The coronary ostia are often stenosed and there is considerable widening of the commissures of the aortic valve with thickening of the valve leaflets. The endarteric process leads to loss of elastic fibers in the media and fibrosis (Figure 8). The wall is so weakened by this process that dilitation and/or aneurysmal formation occurs (Figure 9). Characteristically this involves the ascending portion of the aorta, although other portions may be involved.

Central nervous system syphilis: There is much evidence to suggest that the central nervous system may be involved in the early infectious stages of syphilis. Signs of meningeal irritation and changes in the cerebrospinal fluid consisting of increased cellular and protein content are evidenced in a large number of cases. However, not all patients progress to true cases of neurosyphilis. **Neurosyphilis** is usually divided into the **meningovascular** and **parenchymatous** forms, the latter including general **paresis** and **tabes dorsalis**.

In **meningovascular syphilis** there is widespread diffuse thickening of the pia-arachnoid and infiltration of its meshes by lymphocytes and plasma cells. The small meningeal vessels show thickening and infiltration of the adventitia by lymphocytes and plasma cells and in many areas intimal proliferation and vessel thrombosis. The resulting lesions in the brain itself are secondary to the obliteration of its vascular supply. The arachnoiditis in some cases can produce obstruction of the foramen of Luschka and Magendie with resulting obstructive hydrocephalus.

The brain in syphilitic **paresis** is characteristically shrunken and firmer than normal and is covered by opaque, thickened pia-arachnoid. There is considerable dilitation

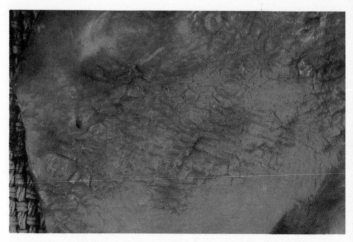

FIGURE 7. Syphilitic aortitis: Markedly irregular and wrinkled intima producing so-called "tree-bark" effect. Several arteriosclerotic plaques are also present.

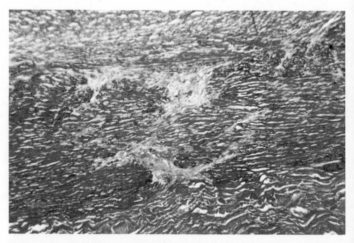

FIGURE 8. Syphilitic aortitis: 450× Elastic stain. The elastic fibers in the media are swollen, irregular and fragmented. A fibrous plaque is replacing the elastic fibers in one area.

30

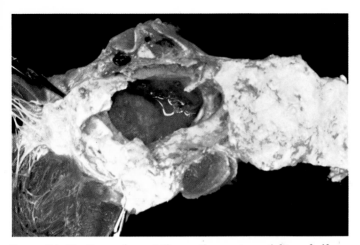

FIGURE 9. Cardiovascular syphilis—aortic aneurysm: A large, fusiform aneurysm involves the ascending portion of the aorta. Rupture has occurred and there is a laminated clot between the media and adventitia. Note the pearly white wrinkled intima in areas distal to the aneurysm.

of the lateral ventricles. The ependyma, especially of the frontal horns and the 3rd and 4th ventricles, shows a coarsely granular appearance. On microscopic examination there is loss of the cortical architecture so that the different layers of the gray matter cannot be easily distinguished. This is due to the loss of numerous neurons, shrinkage and degeneration of other neurons, and an increase in the number of astrocytes and microglia cells. The small blood vessels show thickened walls and many are cuffed by large numbers of plasma cells. The changes in the microglia are extremely characteristic. The bipolar forms are oriented perpendicularly to the surface, and have proliferated and become greatly elongated. This form of microglia is called a **rod cell** and is especially characteristic of the paretic brain (Figure 10). *Treponema pallidum* is identified in this form of neurosyphilis by special stains (Figure 11).

The lesion in **tabes dorsalis** is characteristically concen-

31

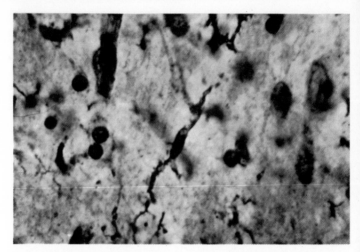

FIGURE 10. CNS syphilis—general paresis: 950× Hortega Silver stain. Bipolar, elongated microglia or rod cells characteristic of general paresis.

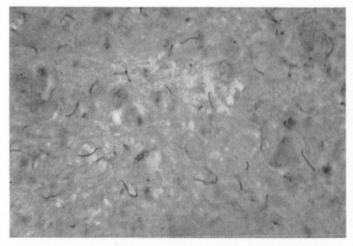

FIGURE 11. CNS syphilis—general paresis: 950× Silver stain. Numerous treponemes identified by silver impregnation technique.

trated in the dorsal roots and in columns of the spinal cord at the lumbosacral and lower thoracic areas. Gross examination of the spinal cord shows diffuse meningeal thickening. This is greater over the dorsal than over the ventral surface of the cord. The cord is somewhat flattened due to shrinkage of the dorsal columns, which on cut section appear gray throughout their width, especially in the lower part of the cord. In sections stained for myelin there is rather diffuse demyelinization of the posterior columns and degeneration of the dorsal roots (Figure 12). In addition there is diffuse lymphocytic and plasma cell infiltration of the leptomeninges of the cord.

Syphilitic **optic atrophy** may be looked upon as a form of neurosyphilis, or as closely associated with neurosyphilis (Figure 13). The optic atrophy may be produced in one of several ways. Syphilitic hydrocephalus or cerebral gummas may interrupt or bring about the distintegration of the optic

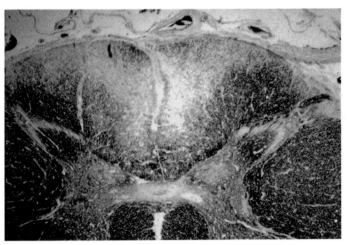

FIGURE 12. CNS syphilis—tabes dorsalis: 450✕ Myelin stain. There is severe demyelinization of the posterior columns.

nerve or optic radiations, thus resulting in blindness. In addition the arachnoid covering the optic nerve may become involved by a fulminating arachnoiditis, producing degeneration of the nerve and resultant blindness. Classical primary optic atrophy of syphilis is most often associated with tabes dorsalis. The lesion is thought to be due to chronic inflammation of the pia matter in the endocranial part of the optic nerve and in the chiasma. Microscopically lymphocytic and plasma cell exudate with fibrous thickening of the meninges can be found. In many cases treponemes can be identified in the sheath of the optic nerves. The exact pathogenesis of primary optic atrophy has not as yet been elucidated.

Congenital syphilis: While the diagnosis of early congenital syphilis may be somewhat difficult, a combination of history, serological findings, and pathological examina-

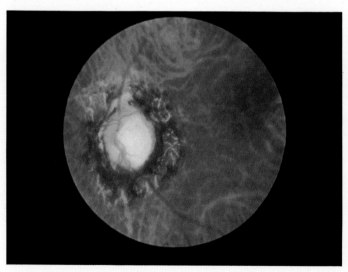

FIGURE 13. Severe optic atrophy and chorioretinitis resulting from late neuro-ocular syphilis.

tion usually establishes a correct diagnosis. While there is nothing particularly characteristic about the widespread organ fibrosis and extramedullary hematopoiesis occurring in the liver and spleen, rather characteristic findings are encountered in the placenta, the bones, and the lungs. In congenital syphilis the placenta is larger, more thickened, and paler than normal. The pale color is caused by the larger size of the villi in relation to the amount of blood in the capillaries. Microscopic examination reveals enlarged villi with bullous projections. The stroma is made up of dense connective tissue. The capillaries are distributed throughout the substance of the villi and are surrounded by a considerable increase in connective tissue (Figure 14). In addition, plasma cells and lymphocytes may be present. *Treponema pallidum* can frequently be demonstrated with appropriate stains. The osseous lesions in congenital syphilis

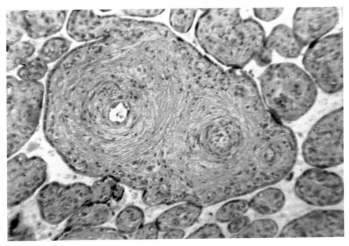

FIGURE 14. Congenital syphilis—placenta: 450× H&E stain. The chorionic villi are enlarged and contain dense laminated connective tissue. The capillaries distributed throughout the villi are compressed by the connective tissue proliferation.

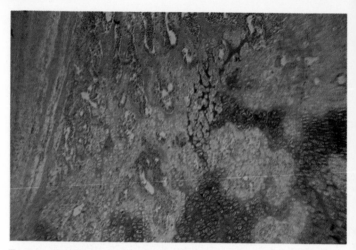

FIGURE 15. Congenital syphilis—osteochondritis: 100× H&E stain. Marked irregularity in the provisional zone of ossification, producing a "sawtoothed" appearance. Note small islands of cartilage remaining in the ossified bone.

include osteochondritis and periostitis. The long bones of the extremities and the ribs are usually the most severely involved. Gross examination of the longitudinally cut section of bone shows an irregular jagged line measuring 1 to 2 mm. in diameter interposed between bone and cartilage. Histologic study shows irregular ingrowth of capillaries with corresponding irregularity in the provisional zone of calcification. This produces the characteristic "sawtoothed" appearance visible both grossly and on roentgen examination. Small isolated groups of undestroyed cartilage cells may remain in the juxta-epiphyseal portion of the metaphasis (Figure 15). The periostitis is characterized by a subperiosteal deposit of osteoid which may completely encircle the shaft of the long bone. It is not incorporated into the shaft, but remains a distinct layer which can be readily observed by roentgen study. With adequate treatment these

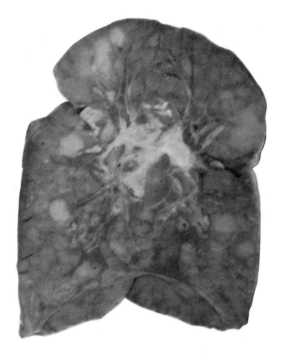

FIGURE 16. Congenital syphilis—pneumonia alba: The lungs are enlarged, heavy, uniformly firm, and yellow-white in color.

changes disappear rather promptly. The lung affected by congenital syphilis results in the so-called pneumonia alba. These lungs are grossly enlarged, heavy, uniformly firm, and yellow-white (Figure 16). The increased weight and density result from distention of the alveoli and alveolar ducts by microphages and from an increase in the connective tissue in the interalveolar septa. Alveoli may have failed to develop and may be completely absent in an infant at term (Figure 17). The pulmonary tree is then composed only of bronchi and alveolar ducts. Polymorphonuclear leukocytes may be present, but the predominant cells of the exudate are usually mononuclear.

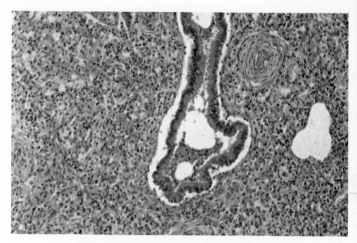

FIGURE 17. Congenital syphilis—pneumonia alba: 100× H&E stain. An alveolar duct is seen in the center. The alveoli are poorly developed and have markedly thickened walls. Macrophages are present in the alveolar spaces.

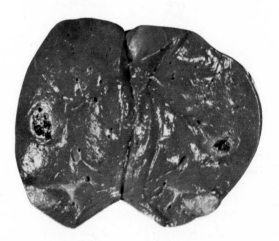

FIGURE 18. Gummas—liver: Two gummas are seen in this specimen. At the lower periphery one is seen as a firm, white, somewhat irregular nodule. The other is hemorrhagic and largely necrotic.

38

Late benign syphilis: The gumma is the hallmark of the lesions of late benign syphilis and a classic example of granulomatous inflammation. The gumma may occur in any organ or tissue of the body and it should be emphasized that when the lesion occurs in such essential organs as the brain or heart, the condition may well not be "benign." The gumma grossly is a firm white lesion which may vary from microscopic size to 10 cm. or more in diameter (Figure 18). Grossly, they may frequently be confused with neoplasms. Histologically the gumma consists of an area of caseous necrosis surrounded by large numbers of lymphocytes, plasma cells, and vascular proliferation showing a characteristic perivascular infiltrate. This latter criteria, particularly, helps to distinguish this lesion from the tubercle as seen in tuberculosis. Giant cells may be present but they are not so numerous as in tuberculosis. *Treponema pallidum* is only rarely found in gummatous lesions.

Bibliography

1. ANDERSON, WILLIAM A. D.: Pathology. Fifth Edition. St. Louis, C. V. Mosby Company, 1966.
2. BREED, ROBERT S.; MURRAY, E. G. D., AND SMITH, NATHAN R.: Bergey's Manual of Determinative Bacteriology. Seventh Edition. Baltimore, The Williams & Wilkins Company, 1957.
3. GREENFIELD, JOSEPH G.: Neuropathology. First Edition. London, Edward Arnold Ltd., 1960.
4. LEVER, WALTER F.: Histopathology of the Skin. Third Edition. Philadelphia, J. B. Lippincott, 1961.
5. POTTER, EDITH L.: Pathology of the Fetus and the Newborn. Chicago, The Year Book Publishers, 1952.
6. TURNER, THOMAS BOURNE, AND HOLLANDER, DAVID H.: Biology of the Treponematoses. Geneva, Switzerland, World Health Organization, 1957.

7. WILLCOX, RICHARD R.: A Textbook of Venereal Diseases and Treponematoses. Second Edition. Springfield, Ill., Charles C. Thomas, 1964.

8. WILLCOX, R. R., AND GUTHE, T.: *Treponema pallidum*— A Bibliographical Review of the Morphology, Culture and Survival of *T. pallidum* and Associated Organisms. Supplement to Volume 35 of the Bull. World Health Organ., Geneva, Switzerland, 1966.

9. ZINSSER, HANS: Microbiology. Thirteenth Edition. New York, Appleton-Century-Crofts, Inc., 1964.

Chapter III.—CLINICAL DIAGNOSIS
OF SYPHILIS

Prior to the 1940's most physicians were well trained in didactic syphilology and had the opportunity to observe many clinical cases. However, those receiving formal education within the past 15-20 years are lucky to have been exposed to even a few hours of syphilology; and exceptional has been their experience if they have ever seen more than a few cases of syphilis. As a consequence, many physicians have been graduated without an adequate knowledge of the many faces of syphilis. Without a high index of suspicion on the part of the physician this "great imitator" will go undiagnosed and continue its path of destruction.

This book does not pretend to be an exhaustive text on the subject of syphilis. It is an attempt to provide the physician with a set of sound guidelines and a few rules of thumb which will give him confidence and expedite his decisions in the diagnosis and treatment of this disease. It is also intended to show that there are no isolated cases of infectious syphilis but that every case of primary and secondary syphilis is directly related to at least one additional case, and that careful exploitation in the area of epidemiology must be carried out with a sense of immediacy.

History and Physical Examination

An accurate history is important and often essential to the diagnosis and treatment of syphilis. In obtaining the history one should speak the language of the layman. The routine medical history should include chief complaint, present illness, past and social history, and review of systems. Such a history should include information on:

Previous infection (memory of "Bad Blood", "Lues" or "Hair Cut", or other venereal disease).

Remembered signs and symptoms (all prior lesions of the skin and genitalia, eye complaints, sore throat, rash, hair loss, etc.).

Parental or family infection (blood tests, illness, miscarriages, stillbirths, etc.).

Previous serologic tests (premarital, prenatal, military, employment, hospitalization, food-handler) and lumbar puncture.

Treatment which might have been antisyphilitic (memory of "hip and arm" shots).

Recent antibiotics (given for ailments other than syphilis). Drug reactions.

The necessity of a careful and complete physical examination, including neurological evaluation and a routine serologic test for syphilis, cannot be overstressed. The patient should be completely unclothed when conducting this examination. All cutaneous surfaces, including the mucous membranes and anogenital region, must be examined in good light, preferably daylight. Other valuable procedures, which may be indicated, depending on the individual case, include chest fluoroscopy or roentgen examination of the chest, darkfield examination of the lesion, confirmatory serologic tests for syphilis, and spinal fluid examination.

Darkfield Examination

Because *Treponema pallidum* is not stained readily by ordinary laboratory methods and is so similar to other spirochetes which inhabit the mouth and genitalia of non-syphilitic persons, it is essential that the organism be seen in the living state. Because of the narrow width of *T. pallidum* the ordinary light microscope does not permit sufficient resolution to visualize the organism. However, this can be accomplished by the use of darkfield microscopy.

The technique is not difficult, but differentiation of *T. pallidum* from other spiral organisms requires careful study and considerable experience.

T. pallidum is demonstrably present in accessible lesions only during the early stages of syphilis. It is essential, however, that a search for *T. pallidum* be made whenever there is any suspicion that a given lesion, whether of the genitalia, skin or mucous membrane, may be syphilitic.

In collecting specimens for examination, plastic or rubber gloves should be worn to protect the examiner from accidental infection. The surface of the suspected lesion should be cleansed carefully with physiologic saline, dried, and then gently abraded to the point of bleeding. Gentle pressure should be maintained upon the lesion until only clear serum exudes. To increase the exudation of serum, the base of the lesion may be squeezed gently, or suction applied. A drop of the serum is picked up directly on the surface of a glass slide and a cover slip placed over it. Examination under a properly adjusted darkfield microscope is then performed. If there is to be any appreciable delay in examining the specimen, the edges of the cover slips should be coated with petroleum jelly.

The darkfield microscope differs from other microscopes chiefly in use of a darkfield condenser which blocks out the central rays of light and directs the peripheral rays from the side upon the microscopic object under study. Under these conditions light does not enter the microscope objective directly, but only those rays which are reflected upward by the object pass into the eyepiece. The subject thus appears bright against a black background, just as dust particles in the atmosphere become visible when a ray of sunlight enters a darkened room.

T. pallidum can be identified by its morphologic characteristics and by its characteristic motions. These motions consist of a slow forward and backward movement, rotation about the long axis like a corkscrew, and a slight

43

bending, twisting or undulation from side to side. Care must be exercised in the interpretation of positive darkfield examinations from the mouth or moist areas of the genitalia since saprophytic spirochetes from these areas may be morphologically identical with *T. pallidum.*

Failure to demonstrate the organisms from the suspected lesion after repeated properly performed examinations may mean that the lesion is not syphilitic; the patient has received systemic or local treatment; too much time has elapsed since the appearance of the lesion; or the lesion may be a late manifestation of syphilis.

Spinal Fluid Examination

The only means of diagnosing neurosyphilis accurately and evaluating its treatment is by spinal fluid examination. Not infrequently neurosyphilis can be demonstrated months or years before the development of subjective or objective neurologic evidence of the disease. For this reason examination of the cerebrospinal fluid should be part of the management in every case of syphilis. In early forms of the disease the examination is most meaningful 6 months to 1 year after treatment; in latent or late forms of the disease examination should precede treatment. A diagnosis of latent syphilis cannot be made unless asymptomatic neurosyphilis is excluded by a negative cerebrospinal fluid. (See "Examination of the Spinal Fluid in Neurosyphilis," page 79).

Bibliography

1. BEERMAN, HERMAN: Syphilis. In Current Diagnosis, edited by Howard F. Conn, Robert J. Clohecy, and Rex B. Conn, Jr. Philadelphia, W. B. Saunders Co., 1966.
2. Darkfield Microscopy for the Detection and Identification of *Treponema Pallidum.* PHS Publ. 990. Washington, D.C., U.S. Government Printing Office, 1962.

Chapter IV.—PRIMARY SYPHILIS

Clinical Signs

The first clinical sign of syphilis is the chancre. Anywhere from 10 to 90 days (average 21 days) following infection, a sore or chancre develops at the site where treponemal invasion occurred (Figures 19 and 20). Certain clinical characteristics assist in arriving at the correct diagnosis, but it should be remembered that frequently the clinical picture is highly atypical and all genital or anal lesions are suspect until proven otherwise.

Chancres are usually single lesions, but multiple lesions are not rare (Figures 21 and 22). The lesion is usually an eroded papule that is decidedly firm and indurated. The surface may be crusted or ulcerated. The size varies from a few millimeters in diameter (Figure 23) to 1 or 2 centimeters (Figures 24, 25 and 26). The border surrounding the lesion is frequently raised and firm. When free of other infectious agents the chancre is typically painless. However, extragenital chancres may be painful. Lymphatic glands draining the involved area are frequently enlarged, hard, and painless (satellite bubo). Genital lesions in males due to syphilis will usually show bilateral lymphadenopathy. Darkfield examination of fluid obtained by needle aspiration of a bubo can be diagnostic in cases where sufficient fluid cannot be obtained from the chancre itself, where the patient has applied topical medications to his lesion, or where the chancre is hidden under a phimotic foreskin or within the urethra. Genital chancres are observed much less frequently in women because of their location within

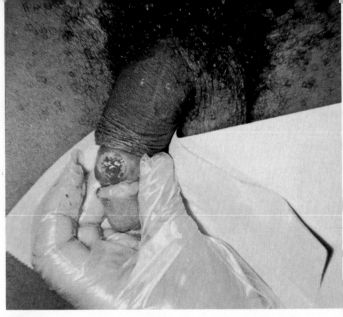

FIGURE 19. Primary syphilis: Typical chancre located at coronal sulcus.

FIGURE 20. Primary syphilis: Chancre of fourchette.

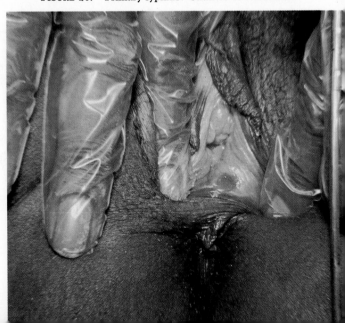

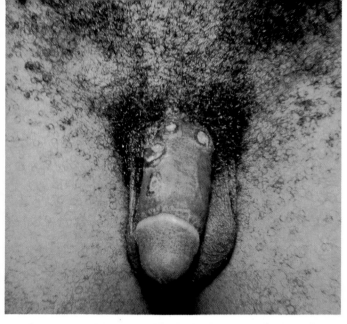

FIGURE 21.   Primary syphilis: Multiple primary chancres of penile shaft.

FIGURE 22.   Primary syphilis: Multiple primary chancres of the labium minora.

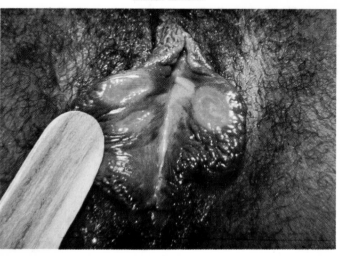

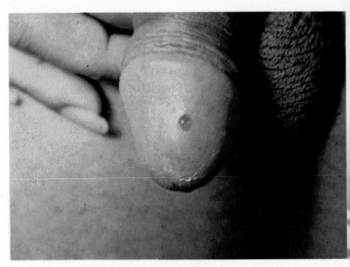

FIGURE 23. Primary syphilis: Small atypical darkfield positive chancre of the glans.

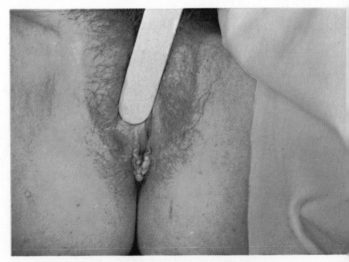

FIGURE 24. Primary syphilis: Vulvar chancre and condylomata acuminata.

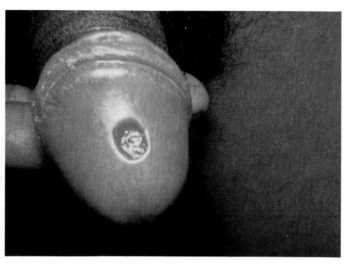

FIGURE 25. Primary syphilis: Chancre of the glans.

FIGURE 26. Primary syphilis: Meatal chancre.

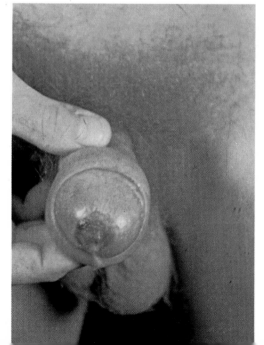

the vagina or on the cervix (Figure 27), although some chancres may be seen on the labia. Careful examination with a speculum is essential to detect these lesions. On the cervix the clinical appearance may vary from an erosion to a deep ulceration resembling carcinoma.

Primary lesions are not confined to the genitalia, and extragenital chancres may be seen on the lips, tongue, tonsil, nipple, fingers, and anus (Figures 28 and 29). In recent years the latter site has become increasingly recognized as due to homosexual transmission. Even without treatment the chancre will heal completely within a 4 to 6 week period. The longer the chancre has been present, the greater the likelihood that serologic tests will be reactive. If the lesion has been present a month, nearly all reagin tests will be reactive.

The possibility of syphilis must be considered when a genital lesion is present, and a darkfield must be performed. If the initial examination is negative, highly suspicious

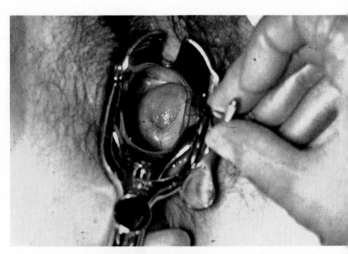

FIGURE 27. Primary syphilis: Primary lesion of cervical os.

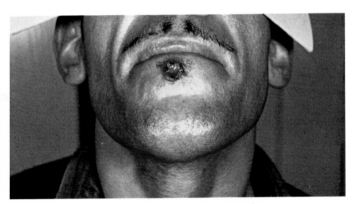

FIGURE 28.   Primary syphilis: Typical Hunterian chancre on lower lip.

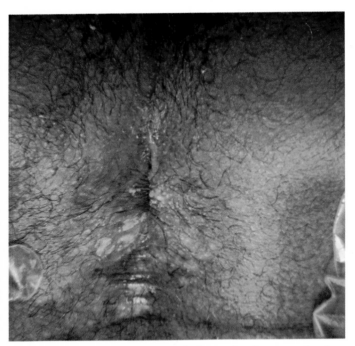

FIGURE 29.   Primary syphilis: Anal chancre in a homosexual male.

51

lesions should have repeated darkfield examinations on successive days before syphilis can be ruled out. Serologic tests should be taken at the time of darkfield examination and repeated at weekly intervals for a month or more until syphilis or a different diagnosis is established.

If a genital lesion is healing, a presumptive diagnosis can be made without a confirmatory darkfield in the presence of lymphadenopathy, a reactive serologic test, and a history of sexual exposure to an infected individual.

Differential Diagnosis of Primary Syphilis

In the differential diagnosis of *any genital lesion primary syphilis should be considered as suspect until ruled out clinically and by specific procedures.*

The following diseases or conditions may suggest primary syphilis, but may be differentiated by some of the indicated criteria:

FIGURE 30. Differential diagnosis: Chancroidal ulcers.

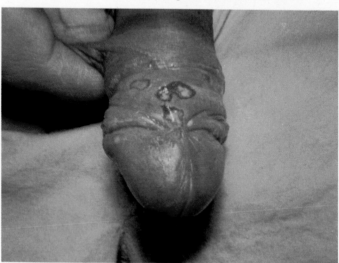

Chancroid—The lesions are usually multiple, soft, tender erosions or ulcerations with a grayish base (Figure 30). Both the lesions and the associated adenopathy, often more pronounced on one side, are quite painful. Darkfield examination is negative. *H. ducreyi* may be demonstrated from the lesion by direct stained smear or by culture. Occasional chancroid patients will have low-titered false positive serologic tests.

Granuloma inguinale—This disease is characterized by a soft, painless, raised, raw beef-colored, smooth granulating lesion (Figure 31). There is no significant adenopathy, darkfield is negative, and the serologic tests are nonreactive. The pathognomonic Donovan bodies *(Donovania granulomatis)* are best demonstrated by direct tissue spread smears stained with hematological dyes such as Wright's stain. Biopsy may demonstrate the causative organisms and rule out carcinoma.

FIGURE 31. Differential diagnosis: Granuloma inguinale with both active and healed areas.

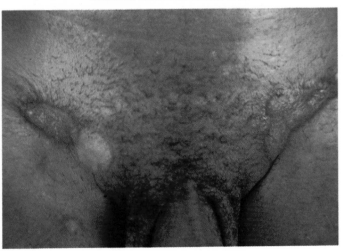

Lymphogranuloma venereum—The initial lesion is a small, transient, rarely seen vesiculo-ulcer. The patient usually shows unilateral, painful, inguinal adenopathy. *Treponema pallidum, Donovania granulomatis,* and *Hemophilus ducreyi* are all excluded by specific studies. A rising titer as detected by complement fixation tests against the causative organism, *Bedsonia lymphogranulomatic,* is diagnostic.

Herpes progenitalis—This viral process is usually manifested by grouped painful, vesicular lesions. History usually reveals recurrent lesions at the same site. The smear technique demonstrates typical viral "balloon" cells. This virus is easily isolated directly from lesions where this laboratory service is available.

Carcinoma—Usually the lesion has been present for a considerable period. The diagnosis is established by biopsy of any suspicious fungating or infiltrating ulcerative lesion.

Scabies—Pruritic vesicles with burrow formation are highly suggestive. Finding the mite in the burrow is diagnostic. The burrow may provide a break in the skin for inoculation with *T. pallidum.*

Trauma—Here a history of injury is usual. The darkfield is negative and serologic tests for syphilis are nonreactive.

Lichen planus—Genital lesions are usually annular or the typical polygonal, flat-topped, violaceous papules. They may be pruritic and may be single or multiple. Serologic tests for syphilis are nonreactive.

Psoriasis—This disease often presents an erythematous or erythemato-squamous plaque on the glans. Removal of the scale produces pinpoint bleeding. Serologic tests for syphilis are nonreactive.

Drug eruptions—One site of predilection of a "fixed" dermatitis medicamentosa is the genital region. Antipyrine, phenolphthalein, phenacetin, barbiturates, salicylates, sulfonamides, and antibiotics are among the most common causes. Careful inquiry as to drug ingestion is imperative. Serologic tests for syphilis are usually nonreactive.

Aphthosis—This condition presents as round to polycyclic, painful, mucous membrane erosions frequently occurring in association with pseudomembranous oral inflammations and ocular lesions.

Deep mycotic infections—The deep fungi may produce chancriform genital lesions. The diagnosis is confirmed by potassium hydroxide preparations, culture, culture mount, and biopsy. Serologic tests for syphilis are nonreactive.

Reiter's syndrome—This syndrome consists of the triad of nonspecific urethritis, mucopurulent conjunctivitis, and polyarticular arthritis. Superficial lesions of the glans penis, however, may occur and are similar to those of an erosive circinate balanitis. Diagnosis is made clinically and corroborated by biopsy.

While one can make an educated guess on morphologic grounds alone, the definitive diagnosis of primary syphilis can be made or eliminated only by appropriate laboratory tests.

Syphilis can be ruled out by:
1. Darkfield examination studies, combined with:
2. Serologic reagin tests, both qualitative and quantitative, and
3. Specific treponemal tests, particularly the FTA-ABS (see page 105) if the above are equivocable.

In summary it is important to remember that:
1. Many nonvenereal genital diseases mimic primary syphilis.
2. Extragenital chancres are not uncommon.
3. Other venereal (e.g., gonorrhea, chancroid) and non-venereal disease (e.g., lichen planus, scabies, etc.) may coexist with primary syphilis.

55

Bibliography

1. King, Ambrose, and Nicol, Claude: Venereal Diseases. Philadelphia, F. A. Davis Company, 1964.
2. Pariser, Harry: Infectious Syphilis. M. Clin. North America, 48:625-636, May 1964.

Chapter V.—SECONDARY SYPHILIS

Clinical Signs

Secondary syphilis is quite varied in its clinical manifestations and may involve any cutaneous or mucosal surface of the body as well as any organ. Although iritis and constitutional symptoms such as fever and malaise may be present, the diagnosis of secondary syphilis is suspected primarily on the basis of the skin and mucous membrane lesions. The skin lesions are bilaterally symmetrical, and may be macular, papular, follicular, papulosquamous, or pustular (Figures 32 through 42). They are seldom pruritic and are usually dry. Vesiculo-bullous lesions do not occur in adults, but may be seen in neonatal congenital syphilis. In secondary relapsing syphilis, lesions tend to be arciform and may be asymmetrical. "Moth-eaten" scalp alopecia beginning in the occipital hair is characteristic (Figure 43). Loss of the eyelashes and the lateral third of the eyebrows may occur (Figure 44). Moist papules occur most frequently in the ano-genital region (condylomata lata) (Figures 45, 46, and 47) and the mouth, but they may be seen on any body surface where moisture can accumulate between intertriginous surfaces (e.g., axillae or toe webs) (Figure 48). Lesions of the mouth, throat, and cervix (mucous patches) frequently occur in secondary syphilis (Figures 49 through 51). Occasionally secondary lesions occur while the chancre of primary syphilis is still present (Figure 52). An extremely important concomitant finding in secondary syphilis is generalized lymphadenopathy. Splenomegaly is occasionally present.

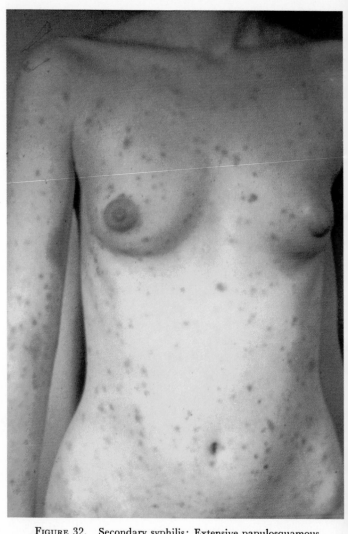

FIGURE 32.   Secondary syphilis: Extensive papulosquamous
rash on body.

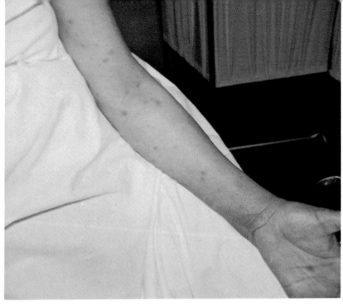

FIGURE 33.   Secondary syphilis: Papular rash on arm and palm.

FIGURE 34.   Secondary syphilis: Papulosquamous lesions of penis, scrotum, and thighs.

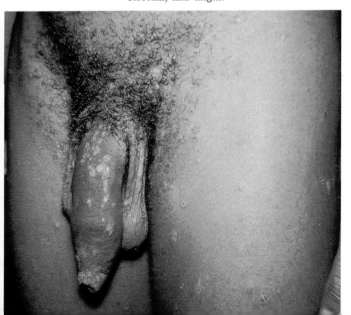

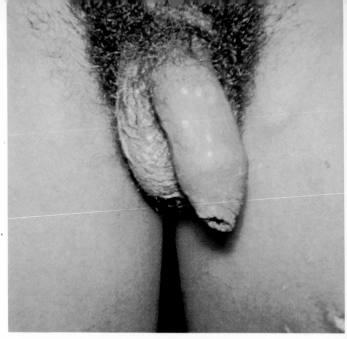

FIGURE 35. Secondary syphilis: Secondary lesions of penis
having psoriasiform appearance.

FIGURE 36. Secondary syphilis: Annular squamous lesions of scrotum.

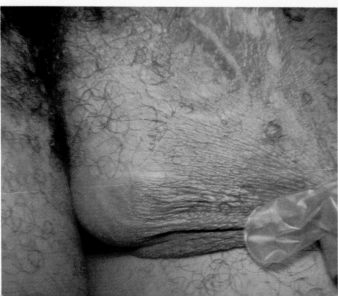

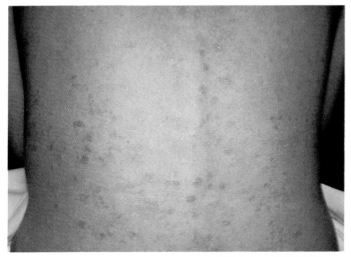

FIGURE 37.   Secondary syphilis: Secondary lesions resembling
pityriasis rosea.

FIGURE 38.   Secondary syphilis: Papulosquamous lesions on
back and shoulder.

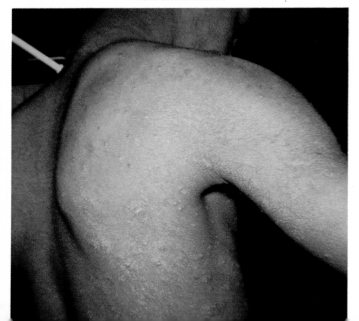

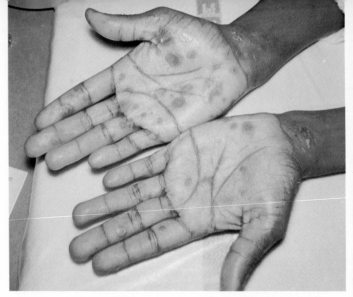

FIGURE 39. Secondary syphilis: Papulosquamous syphilids of wrists and palms.

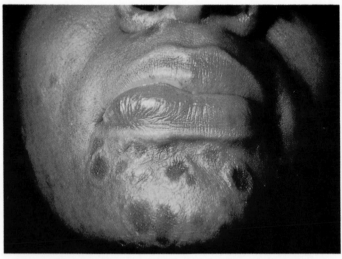

FIGURE 40. Secondary syphilis: Typical "nickel and dime" lesions.

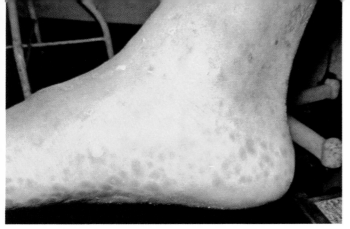

FIGURE 41. Secondary syphilis: Macular syphilids of foot.

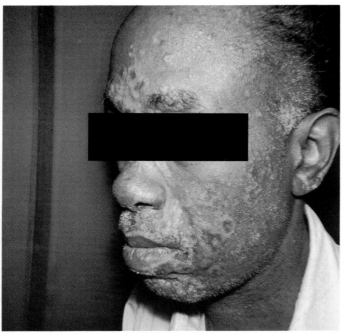

FIGURE 42. Secondary syphilis: Extensive secondary lesions of face.

63

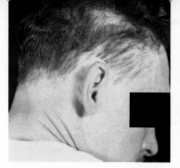

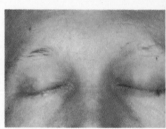

FIGURE 43. Secondary syphilis: Alopecia of scalp in secondary syphilis.

FIGURE 44. Secondary syphilis: Eyebrow alopecia in secondary syphilis.

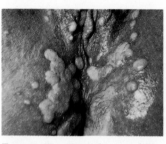

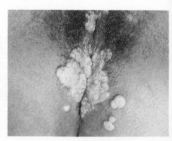

FIGURE 45. Secondary syphilis: Condylomata lata involving vulva and anal region.

FIGURE 46. Secondary syphilis: Anogenital condylomata lata.

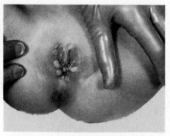

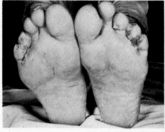

FIGURE 47. Secondary syphilis: Vulvar condylomata lata in child who had been sexually molested.

FIGURE 48. Moist papules developing in the intertriginous areas of the toes.

64

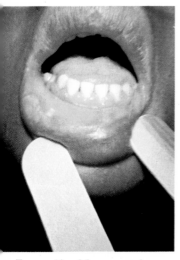

FIGURE 49. Mucous patches
on lower lip.

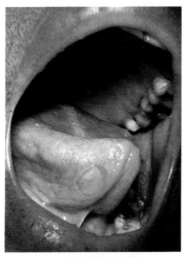

FIGURE 50. Secondary syphilis:
Mucous patch of the tongue.

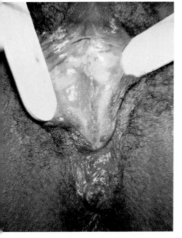

FIGURE 51. Secondary syphilis:
Mucous patches of vestibule.

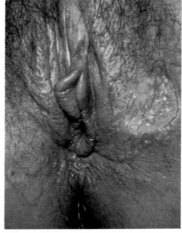

FIGURE 52. Coexistent chancre
and secondary vulvar mucosal lesions.

65

Whenever feasible it is preferable to diagnose secondary syphilis on the basis of a positive darkfield and a reactive serologic test for syphilis. As a rule *Treponema pallidum* may be obtained from any mucous or cutaneous secondary lesions, but most easily from a moist one. Failure to demonstrate *Treponema pallidum* in suspect lesions does not, however, rule out the diagnosis of secondary syphilis. Drying of lesions, imperfect darkfield microscopy, use of topical antibiotic or other creams, local antiseptics, soaps or systemic antibiotics may result in a failure to find diagnostic organisms. For practical purposes the diagnosis may be established without a positive darkfield if characteristic skin and mucous membrane lesions are present and the serologic tests are reactive in high titer. The history of a recent primary lesion is also helpful.

The nontreponemal serologic tests are uniformly reactive during this stage of the disease, and most of the treponemal serologic tests are also reactive. For a discussion of the prozone phenomenon see "Serologic Interpretation," page 102.

Differential Diagnosis of Secondary Syphilis

Pityriasis rosea—Erythematous, maculo-papulosquamous lesions occur along the lines of skin cleavage, which usually spare the distal parts of the extremities, head and neck, and mucous membranes. The body eruption is often preceded for one or more weeks by a single lesion, the herald patch. The darkfield examination is negative, and the serologic tests for syphilis are nonreactive.

Psoriasis—Erythematous, maculo-papulosquamous lesions commonly appear on the scalp, elbows, knees, chest, back, and buttocks. The nails and intertriginous areas may be involved. Manual removal of scales will produce pinpoint areas of bleeding. There is usually a history of chronicity. The darkfield examination is negative, and the serologic tests for syphilis are nonreactive.

Lichen planus—Violaceous, papular, pruritic lesions occur most commonly on wrists, ankles, and sacral areas. Genital and oral lesions may occur, but the darkfield examination is negative for *T. pallidum* and the serologic tests for syphilis are nonreactive.

Tinea veriscolor—Typified by brown, superficial scaly lesions which at times may be erythematous; scrapings for spores and hyphae are positive.

Drug eruptions—Skin lesions are widely varied in their form. They may be macular or bullous; localized or generalized; acute or chronic. A careful history is of utmost importance. The darkfield examination is negative and the serologic tests for syphilis are nonreactive.

"Id" eruptions—Lesions are diversified, but may be papulosquamous, macular, or vesicular. Dermatophyte infection, bacterial infection, and/or eczematous processes are usually demonstrable in other parts of the body. The darkfield examination is negative, and the serologic tests for syphilis are nonreactive.

Perlèche—The fissured split papules which may occur at the angles of the mouth in secondary syphilis mimic the fissuring occasionally associated with cheilitis, hypovitaminosis, and oral moniliasis. Serologic tests for syphilis are negative.

Parasites—Scabies and pediculosis infestations are suggested by excoriated papules and pustules often in intertriginous areas (e.g., finger and toe webs; groin and axillae). Pruritus is severe. The darkfield examination is negative, and the serologic tests for syphilis are nonreactive. Demonstration of the parasite is diagnostic.

Iritis and Neuroretinitis—When these are part of the secondary syphilis syndrome, they are accompanied by other recognizable lesions of secondary syphilis. Some of the serologic tests for syphilis will be reactive.

Condylomata acuminata—These verrucous acuminate lesions, which are of viral origin, may occur in any moist intertriginous area, but are seen most frequently around the glans, vulva, and rectal regions. Darkfield examination may reveal large numbers of saprophytic treponemes, but no *Treponema pallidum*. The serologic tests for syphilis are nonreactive.

Acute exanthemata—Epidemic, generalized, moribilliform, occasionally petechial eruptions associated with fever and constitutional symptoms are the usual manifestations. The darkfield examination is negative, and the serologic tests for syphilis are usually nonreactive. (See "Serologic Interpretation," page 106, with reference to false positive serologic tests for syphilis.)

Infectious mononucleosis—The generalized eruption (present in approximately 10 percent of the cases), lymphadenopathy and inflamed throat closely resemble the symptoms seen in secondary syphilis. Very rarely some of the serologic tests for syphilis are reactive (see "Serologic Interpretation," page 106, with reference to false positive serologic tests for syphilis), and the spleen may be markedly enlarged. Careful darkfield examination of lesions may be necessary to exclude syphilis. Atypical lymphocytes in the blood smear and a positive heterophile agglutination test establish the diagnosis.

Alopecia—The nonscarring temporary hair loss seen in secondary syphilis, described in the opening paragraph of this section, is usually associated with other characteristic cutaneous lesions. The serologic tests for syphilis are uniformly reactive, and darkfield examination of moist lesions occurring elsewhere will be positive for *Treponema pallidum*. Toxic and traumatic alopecia, as well as alopecia areata, may be ruled out by history, examination of the hair, negative darkfield examination, and nonreactive serologic tests for syphilis.

Any of the above conditions can occur concurrently with syphilis.

Bibliography

1. PILLSBURY, DONALD M., SHELLEY, WALTER B., AND KLIGMAN, ALBERT M.: A Manual of Cutaneous Medicine. Philadelphia, W. B. Saunders Co., 1961.
2. STOKES, JOHN H., BEERMAN, HERMAN, AND INGRAHM, NORMAN R., JR., Modern Clinical Syphilology. Third Edition. Philadelphia, W. B. Saunders Co., 1944.
3. SUTTON, RICHARD L.: Diseases of the Skin. Eleventh Edition. St. Louis, C. V. Mosby Company, 1956.
4. Syphilis and Other Venereal Diseases. M. Clin. North America, Vol. 48, No. 3, May 1964.

Chapter VI.—EPIDEMIOLOGY OF SYPHILIS

Every case of infectious syphilis must be considered as suggestive of a potential epidemic. Since no case occurs in isolation, it must be remembered that the disease exists because a personal interchange of the infecting organism took place through some form of intimate physical contact with another person. These facts necessarily indicate that any control procedures must take into account medical as well as social considerations and both normal and deviate behavior.

Syphilis epidemiology is simple in theory, but complex in application. The busy physician will find it difficult, if not impossible, to involve himself in this demanding and time consuming process.

All state health departments, and most local health units, have specially trained personnel who are able to skillfully handle the great variety of personal and social problems related to sexual behavior and venereal disease. They are schooled in interviewing and investigation techniques which ensure confidentiality and bring to treatment the maximum number of infected contacts.

The epidemiology of infectious syphilis revolves around an organized set of techniques which have produced desired results when carried out with maximum speed and thoroughness. The following discussion outlines the basic procedure for applied syphilis epidemiology.

Patient Interview

An interview should be performed promptly upon diagnosis for the purpose of eliciting not only sexual contacts but also a select group of persons known by the original patient as syphilis suspects or associates. In addition, the interview must serve as an information-giving process to inform the patient about his disease.

Each case of syphilis must receive individual consideration preparatory to interviewing, based upon the available medical and epidemiologic information. As a rule, however, primary syphilis cases should be interviewed to elicit sexual contacts during the three months prior to the onset of symptoms. Secondary syphilis patients should be interviewed for contact information for the six months prior to the onset of symptoms. Early latent syphilis cases are generally interviewed for the preceding 12 months. The exact interview period will be determined by examining the available medical and epidemiologic information. For every case of syphilis there must be a source contact. If all such named contacts are examined and found not to be infected then the interview is incomplete.

Contact Tracing

In rare instances, a patient with infectious syphilis may have had no additional contact since the beginning of his or her incubation period; this, however, is most unusual. The average patient may be expected to name three or four persons, and it is not unusual for a greater number of contacts to be involved. Any one of these contacts not found and examined may develop the disease, pass it on to other persons, and later become afflicted with the damaging late manifestations.

The mobility of our population makes it imperative that the exchange of contact information between geographic areas be accomplished rapidly to ensure prompt examination and treatment of infected contacts. Also it is important that those contacts located and found to be not infected at the time of first examination be given prophylactic (epi-

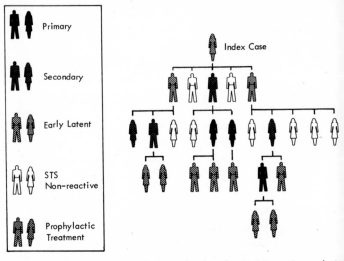

The index case was brought to medical attention through a routine reactive serologic test. Prophylactic treatment was administered to all named sexual contacts who were clinically negative and serologically non-reactive on initial examination, but who were within the critical 90 day incubation period following exposure.

FIGURE 53. The arrest of a syphilis outbreak through prophylactic treatment.

demiologic or preventive) treatment (Figure 53). (See "Prophylactic Treatment," page 115).

If the patient is known to have been exposed to lesion syphilis, it is a fallacy to wait for the disease to develop to the clinical or reactive serologic stage, meanwhile allow ing reinfection of treated patients and the infection of addi tional persons.

In the state and local health departments where epi demiologic assistance is available, more and more physician are using these services. Where these services are not readil available, the physician must make every effort to initiat his own epidemiology on an immediate basis and call upo the state health department for continued assistance.

Bibliography

1. DAVIS, WARREN T., JR.: Epidemiology—the key to vene-real syphilis control. In Proc. World Forum on Syphilis and Other Treponematoses. PHS Publ. 997. Washington, D.C., U.S. Government Printing Office, 1964, pages 33-37.

2. DOUGHERTY, WILLIAM J.: Epidemiologic treatment of syphilis contacts. J. M. Soc. New Jersey, 59:564-567, November 1962.

3. FRYE, WILLIAM W.: The importance of contact investigation in the control of syphilis. M. Clin. North America, 48:637-651, May 1964.

4. KAMPMEIER, RUDOLPH H.: Responsibility of a physician in a program for syphilis eradication. In Proc. World Forum on Syphilis and Other Treponematoses. PHS Publ. 997. Washington, D.C., U.S. Government Printing Office, 1964, pages 70-79.

Chapter VII.—LATENT AND LATE SYPHILIS

Latent Syphilis

By definition latent syphilis is that stage of syphilis where there are no clinical signs or symptoms of the disease; the spinal fluid has been examined and is negative; and serologic tests for syphilis are reactive. All syphilis is latent at some time during its course, and some cases may be virtually latent for the duration of the disease or the life of the patient. A clinical diagnosis of latency does not preclude the possibility of infectiousness, or of developing gummatous lesions, cardiovascular abnormalities, or of neurosyphilis, as yet not apparent. When any of the aforementioned conditions become apparent the diagnosis is no longer latent syphilis.

Syphilis should be diagnosed as latent only after careful history and physical examination have disclosed no abnormalities of syphilitic origin, and the spinal fluid has been shown to be normal.

The diagnosis of latent syphilis is made on the basis of repeated serologic tests in the absence of concurrent disease which may produce a false positive reaction. A treponemal test is often indicated to establish the syphilitic nature of the serologic test reactivity.

A history of exposure, of early lesions, of previous reactive serologic tests, or of antecedent treatment is helpful if elicited, and may help in classification as early or late.

After an infection with syphilis has persisted for more than 4 years, it is rarely communicable, except in the case of the pregnant woman, who if untreated, may transmit syphilis to the fetus, regardless of the duration of her disease. Also, if after 4 years of infection the spinal fluid is normal, in all probability it will remain so.

Late Syphilis

Syphilis is essentially a vascular disease from beginning to end, with the exception of the gumma, which is probably a hyperimmune phenomenon. Aside from gummas the lesions of late syphilis are produced by obliterative endarteritis of terminal arterioles and small arteries, and by the resulting inflammatory and necrotic changes.

As indicated in Table 1, there are practical differentiations in the lesions of early and late syphilis:

TABLE 1

Characteristic	Early Syphilis	Late Syphilis
Infectivity.	Yes.	No, except in pregnant female.
Darkfield.	Positive.	Negative.
Reinfection.	Can occur, after adequate treatment.	Rare, even after adequate treatment.
Destructive lesions.	No.	Yes.
Serologic tests.	Reactive, often with high titer, reverting to negative, or with marked fall to low titer, after treatment.	Usually reactive, often with low titer, with little or no change after treatment. High titers are frequently associated with gummas and paresis.

Untreated late syphilis may present a tremendous range of signs and symptoms, varying from none apparent to those indicating severe damage to one or more body systems. The most usual types of late syphilis, and the chances of their occurrence are:

Type of Late Syphilis	Frequency (percent)
Latent	60–70
Neurosyphilis (Symptomatic)	8
Late Benign Syphilis	17
Cardiovascular Syphilis	10

These divisions of late syphilis are not mutually exclusive. A patient may have more than one type of late involvement; for example:

Of patients with late benign syphilis, about 13 percent will have cardiovascular involvement, and another 10 percent neurosyphilis.

Of patients with cardiovascular syphilis, about 12 percent have associated neurosyphilis.

Of patients with neurosyphilis, about 15 percent have associated cardiovascular syphilis.

Neurosyphilis

All neurosyphilis is asymptomatic at some time during its course, and it is rare for neurosyphilis to occur in "pure" forms. In all types of neurosyphilis the essential changes are the same: obliterative endarteritis, usually of terminal vessels, with associated parenchymatous degeneration which may or may not be sufficient to produce symptoms at the time of examination.

Neurosyphilis is somewhat arbitrarily divided into the following types of groups, which depend on the type and degree of central nervous system pathology present: Asymptomatic; meningovascular; and parenchymatous, consisting of paresis and tabes dorsalis.

Asymptomatic Neurosyphilis—The patient is usually seen because of a reactive serologic test for syphilis. There are no signs or symptoms indicative of central nervous system involvement. Examination of the cerebrospinal fluid is abnormal, with an increase in cells, total protein, and with a reactive VDRL, or Kolmer complement fixation test.

Meningovascular Neurosyphilis—There are definite signs and symptoms of central nervous system damage, which result from cerebral vascular occlusion, infarction, and encephalomalacia with focal neurologic signs varying according to the size and location of the lesion. The cerebrospinal fluid is always abnormal, with an increase in cells, in protein, and showing a reactive VDRL or complement fixation reaction.

Parenchymatous Neurosyphilis—Parenchymatous neurosyphilis presents as paresis or tabes dorsalis:

PARESIS: The signs and symptoms of paresis may be myriad, but are always indicative of widespread parenchymatous damage. Personality changes range from minor to frankly psychotic. Frequently there are focal neurologic signs. The cerebrospinal fluid is invariably abnormal. The VDRL or complement fixation test is reactive and cells and protein are increased. Serologic tests (blood) are reactive.

TABES DORSALIS: The prime signs and symptoms of tabes dorsalis are those of posterior column degeneration, with ataxia, areflexia, paraesthesias, bladder disturbances, impotency, and often, lancinating pain (lightning pains). The spinal fluid findings are abnormal in 90 percent of cases; the blood serology is reactive in 75 percent. Gastric or abdominal "crises" frequently begin with vomiting and severe abdominal pain. Persistent vomiting may cause serious electrolyte imbalance. Trophic joint changes (Charcot's joints) result from the loss or impairment of the sensation of pain. The knee joint is most commonly involved and severe degeneration is common (Figure 54). Similar trophic joint changes may be found in conditions other than syphilis, i.e. syringomyelia, spinal cord injury, or diabetes. The loss of deep pain sensation may be associated with perforating ulcers on the soles or toes (mal perforans) (Figure 55).

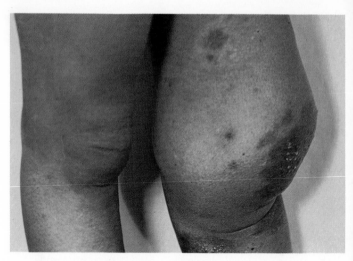

FIGURE 54.   Late syphilis: Charcot knee in tabes dorsalis
of long standing.

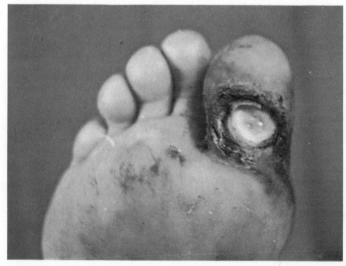

FIGURE 55.   Late syphilis: Perforating ulcer of great toe
(mal perforans) in tabes dorsalis.

Syphilitic optic atrophy is a serious complication of neurosyphilis, and should be looked for in every patient. It is most frequently associated with tabes dorsalis and an examination of peripheral visual fields is imperative in every suspected neurosyphilitic. Pupillary changes may be seen in both forms of late neurosyphilis. The classic Argyll Robertson pupil is small, irregular, and fails to react to light, but reacts normally to convergence. Other pupillary variations from this typical pattern are common.

The signs and symptoms of paresis and tabes dorsalis frequently coexist (so-called taboparesis) in the same patient.

Examination of the Spinal Fluid in Neurosyphilis. — The lumbar puncture can be performed with the subject in the sitting position or placed on his side. In the sitting position, the patient straddles a straight chair, facing the chair back, and arching the spine posteriorly. On his side, the patient arches his back by drawing up the knees and bending the head so that they almost touch. The lumbosacral area should be cleansed with iodine followed by alcohol. A sterile spinal needle is then inserted into the third, fourth, or fifth lumbar interspace and sufficient fluid is collected for study (6-8 ml.). The procedure may be safely performed in the clinic or in the physician's office.

There are three tests of spinal fluid essential for the diagnosis of neurosyphilis, and for its intelligent followup:

1. Cell count: Over 4 lymphocytes is abnormal.

2. Total protein: Protein is always elevated in active neurosyphilis. "Normal" values vary from laboratory to laboratory, depending on the test used. Know your laboratory, and its readings of normal limits. Individuals vary considerably in their normal total protein values, but a total protein of more than 40 mg% is usually abnormal.

3. Kolmer or VDRL spinal fluid tests: A reactive spinal fluid Kolmer or VDRL is practically always an

indication of central nervous system syphilis, but not necessarily of its activity. False positive reactions in the spinal fluid are **rare.**

The presence of reagin in the spinal fluid is the only finding which is pathognomonic of neurosyphilis since any condition which causes meningeal irritation may result in an increase in the cell count and protein concentration of the spinal fluid. Consequently, reactive tests for syphilitic reagin in the spinal fluid are reliable evidence of past or present neurosyphilis. With the exception of late tabes dorsalis, the clinical syndrome is rarely so clear cut as to permit the diagnosis of neurosyphilis in the face of negative reagin serologic findings. Conversely, even in the absence of clinical signs or symptoms, a positive reagin test is indicative of asymptomatic neurosyphilis. Following successful treatment and arrest of late neurosyphilis, it may take many years for the spinal fluid reagin test to become nonreactive.

The degree of activity of neurosyphilis is indicated by increased numbers of lymphocytes and increased protein in the spinal fluid. A cell count of more than 4 per cu. mm. is usually abnormal and indicative of an active central nervous system infection. Every effort should be made to perform cell counts as soon as possible and to avoid contamination of the fluid with red cells since leukocytic cells disintegrate quite rapidly at room temperature and erythrocytes inevitably interfere with accurate counting.

In the diagnosis of central nervous system syphilis, beware of the bloody tap. Small quantities of reactive blood serum in spinal fluid can produce a positive Kolmer or VDRL reaction, and red cells may be mistakenly interpreted as white cells.

Increased total protein in association with pleocytosis and reactive spinal fluid reagin is also indicative of active neurosyphilis. Following successful treatment, high total protein values decline slowly, and they may not become normal for a year, or even several years. In general, the cell count may be expected to return first to normal followed by the protein and finally the serologic test. Examples are given in Table 2.

Colloidal tests of spinal fluid such as the colloidal gold test, once widely utilized, are of no diagnostic significance and are not a reliable guide to the activity of neurosyphilis. These tests have no value in the management of neurosyphilis.

TABLE 2. — Typical Serologic and Cerebrospinal Fluid Responses Following Therapy for Neurosyphilis

DAYS AFTER THERAPY	(SERUM) QUANTITATIVE VDRL	CEREBROSPINAL FLUID		
		LYMPHOCYTES (PER MM^3)	PROTEIN (MG %)	VDRL SLIDE
I. Asymptomatic Neurosyphilis				
0	8 dils	143	92	4 dils
93	8 dils	27	83	4 dils
178	4 dils	9	89	4 dils
271	8 dils	—	—	——
347	4 dils	3	54	2 dils
526	4 dils	—	—	——
727	2 dils	4	47	WR 0 dils
929	N	—	—	——
1344	N	0	44	N
II. Symptomatic Neurosyphilis				
4	16 dils	35	64	4 dils
188	8 dils	8	52	4 dils
374	8 dils	4	50	4 dils
505	4 dils	—	—	——
735	8 dils	5	43	4 dils
984	4 dils	—	—	——
1288	4 dils	4	45	2 dils

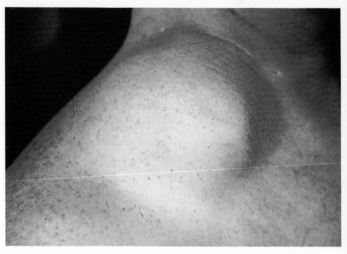

FIGURE 56.   Late syphilis: Aortic aneurysm eroding through ribs and clavicle.

Cardiovascular Syphilis

Cardiovascular syphilis is usually caused by medial necrosis of the aorta, with aortic dilatation which may extend into the valve commissures.

The essential signs of cardiovascular syphilis are those of aortic insufficiency or saccular aneurysm of the thoracic aorta (Figure 56). When fully developed, these conditions are not difficult to detect. Careful clinical evaluation of hypertension, arteriosclerosis, and previous rheumatic heart disease is essential.

Saccular aneurysm of the thoracic aorta is *prima facie* evidence of cardiovascular syphilis; aortic insufficiency with no other valvular lesions in a person of middle age, with a reactive serologic test, should be considered cardiovascular syphilis until proven otherwise.

Serologic tests for syphilis are usually reactive in cardiovascular syphilis.

Late Benign Syphilis

The term "benign" is used because the lesions of late benign syphilis seldom result in total physical incapacity or death, although when such gummas occur in the brain or other vital organs the word "benign" is misleading. The essential lesion of late benign syphilis is the gumma.

Gummas are probably the result of hypersensitivity reactions of treponemal infection. The most common sites are skin, bone and liver, but nearly any organ may be involved.

Skin lesions may be solitary or multiple, tend to form circles or segments of circles, are destructive and chronic, and tend to heal centrally and extend peripherally (Figures 57 through 60).

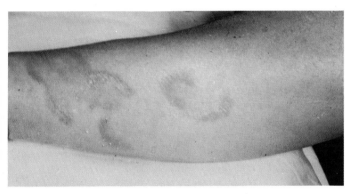

FIGURE 57. Late syphilis: Gummas of the arm.

FIGURE 58. Gummas of the scalp.

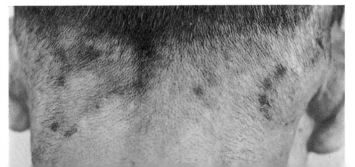

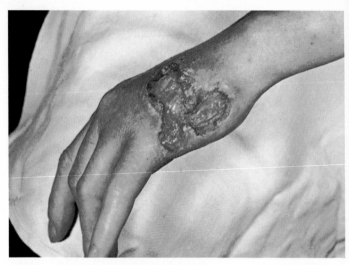

FIGURE 59.　Late syphilis: Gummatous involvement of the hand in late syphilis.

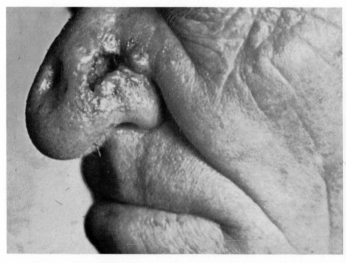

FIGURE 60.　Gummatous involvement of the nose mimicking basal cell carcinoma.

Bone lesions are usually marked by periostitis with associated new bone formation, or by gummatous osteitis, with bone destruction. The cardinal signs are those of pain, swelling, and bony tumor. The most common sites are the cranial bones, the tibia, and the clavicle.

In late benign syphilis, the serologic tests are almost always reactive and usually of **high titer.**

Bibliography

1. BEERMAN, HERMAN AND NICHOLAS, LESLIE: Syphilis. In Volume III, Tice-Harvey Practice of Medicine, pages 329-449. Hagerstown, Md., W. F. Prior Company, Inc., 1964.
2. KAMPMEIER, R. H.: The late manifestations of syphilis; skeletal, visceral and cardiovascular. M. Clin. North America, 48:667-697, May 1964.
3. OLANSKY, SIDNEY: Late benign syphilis (gumma). M. Clin. North America, 48:653-665, May 1964.
4. THOMAS, EVAN W.: Some aspects of neurosyphilis. M. Clin. North America, 48:699-705, May 1964.

Chapter VIII.—SYPHILIS IN PREGNANCY AND CONGENITAL SYPHILIS

After the 18th week of gestation, when the Langhans' cell layer of the early placenta has atrophied, the treponeme may cross the placenta to infect the fetus. A general rule, "Kassowitz' law," is: The longer the duration of the untreated infection before the pregnancy, the less likely it is that the fetus will be stillborn or infected. Thus, pregnancy while the mother is in the primary or secondary stages of infection frequently terminates in a stillbirth, whereas pregnancy occurring during the later stages of syphilis may result in a clinical spectrum from a fulminating fatal congenital syphilis to an uninfected child.

The signs of syphilis which the mother shows will depend on the stage of infection at the time of pregnancy. If the mother becomes infected late in the pregnancy, she may show no signs before delivery and the infected newborn may also appear normal at birth. Syphilis usually causes a stillbirth rather than an abortion, because of the time period in pregnancy when the fetus may first be infected.

Adequate treatment of the mother before the 18th week of pregnancy prevents infection of the fetus. Because penicillin will cross the placenta in adequate amounts, treatment of the mother after the 18th week of pregnancy will also cure the infected fetus. In women who are allergic to penicillin, special precaution must be taken in the selection and dose of the alternative antibiotic (see section on therapy, page 110). A woman who has been adequately treated, and followed with quantitative serologic tests with no evidence of reinfection does not need to be retreated with each subsequent pregnancy.

Congenital syphilis is divided into stages much like the classification of acquired syphilis. However, since the treponeme is introduced directly into the fetal circulation there is no primary stage.

Early Congenital Syphilis

The early stage is characterized by the appearance of signs and symptoms before the age of 2. The earlier the onset in the first few weeks of life usually the poorer the prognosis. These signs may include:

1. *Cutaneous lesions*: The skin lesions seen shortly after birth are frequently vesicular or bullous (as opposed to acquired syphilis in which vesicles are not seen) progressing to superficial crusted erosions. Skin lesions seen in later weeks are frequently papulosquamous with a generalized symmetrical distribution like that of acquired syphilis and may form typical condylomata lata.

2. *Mucous membrane lesions*: The mucous membranes of the nose and pharynx are frequently involved to produce a heavy mucoid discharge which is referred to as "the snuffles." A hemorrhagic nasal discharge in the newborn period is characteristic of syphilis. Both the skin and mucous membrane lesions are teeming with spirochetes, causing these lesions and their secretions to be extremely infectious. A positive diagnosis can be made with darkfield examination. (Figure 61).

3. *Bone*: Involvement usually takes the form of an osteochrondritis of the long bones. Although only 15 percent will show clinical signs, almost 100

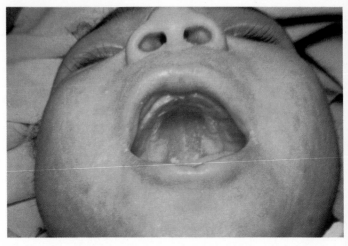

FIGURE 61. Infant demonstrating mucous patches, and skin lesions.

percent will show radiologic changes of this bone involvement after the first month of life. Dactylitis results from involvement of the phalanges.

4. *Anemia*: Most have a hemolytic anemia which is self-limited.

5. *Hepatosplenomegaly*: Frequently present (two-thirds of cases) and may be associated with a low grade icterus.

6. *Central nervous system*: Up to 50 percent may have abnormal cerebrospinal fluid findings; however, the incidence of actual clinical manifestations is much lower.

Late Congenital Syphilis

Late congenital syphilis is defined as congenital syphilis which has persisted beyond 2 years of age. In about 60 percent the disease is latent with no manifestations other than a reactive serologic test for syphilis. The titers of the serologic tests in untreated congenital syphilis may fluctuate greatly, and when such fluctuations are seen this diagnosis should be suspected. The signs of this stage may be produced by continued activity of the disease process or may be the so-called "stigmata" (that is, permanent scars or deformities resulting from previous involvement). Late congenital syphilis is not infectious. The signs of late congenital syphilis may include:

1. *Interstitial keratitis*: Usually appears near puberty and eventually becomes bilateral. The cornea develops a ground glass appearance with vascularization of the adjacent sclera (Figure 62).

2. *Hutchinson's teeth*: Due to the poor development of the middle denticle, the permanent upper (occasionally the lower) central incisors develop a

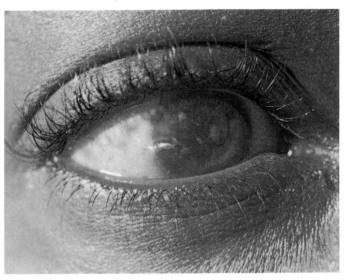

FIGURE 62.   Congenital syphilis: Interstitial keratitis causing blindness.

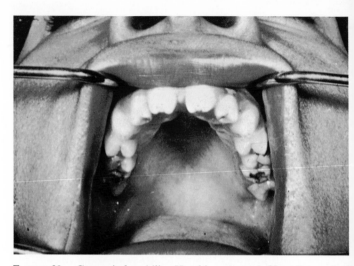

FIGURE 63. Congenital syphilis: Hutchinson's teeth. Note the notched edges and "screwdriver" shape of the central incisors.

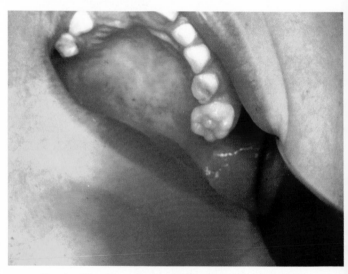

FIGURE 64. Congenital syphilis: Moon's molar of late congenital syphilis.

barrel-shaped and notched appearance and are smaller than normal, causing these teeth to be more widely spaced. Roentgen study of the un-erupted teeth will allow the diagnosis to be made while the uninvolved deciduous teeth are still present (Figure 63).

3. *Mulberry or Moon's molars*: The first molars may show maldevelopment of the cusps (Figure 64).

4. *Eighth nerve deafness*: An unusual manifestation with onset frequently near puberty but occasionally delayed until middle age.

5. *Neurosyphilis*: The congenital syphilitic may show the same manifestations of neurosyphilis as seen in acquired syphilis. Tabes dorsalis is much less common than in the acquired form of the disease; paresis is more frequent than in the adult.

6. *Bone involvement*: This may be sclerotic to produce the sabre shin (Figure 65) and frontal bossing, or it may be lytic (gummatous) and produce destruction, most frequently of the nasal septum (the saddle nose configuration) or the hard palate. Perforation of the palate is very suggestive of congenital syphilis (Figure 66). Any part of the skeletal system may be involved.

7. *Cutaneous involvement*: Rhagades (cracks or fissures about the mouth or nose) may result from infantile syphilitic rhinitis (Figure 67), but are rarely seen. Gummas may involve any portion of the skin or other organ systems as in the acquired form of the disease.

8. *Cardiovascular lesions*: Rare instances of cardiovascular lesions have been reported.

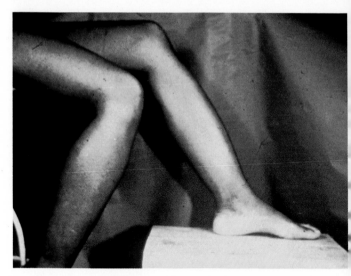

FIGURE 65.   Congenital syphilis: Osteoperiositis of the tibia
resulting in "sabre shins."

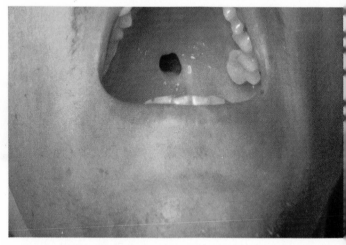

FIGURE 66.   Congenital syphilis: Perforation of hard palate
resulting from gummatous destruction.

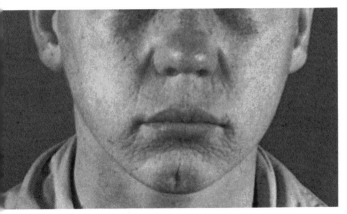

FIGURE 67. Congenital syphilis: "Rhagades" facial disfigurement resulting from persistent syphilitic rhinitis of infancy.

9. *Clutton's joints*: Painless hydroarthrosis, usually of the knees (Figure 68), rarely involving the elbows or other large joints.

Clutton's joints, interstitial keratitis and eighth nerve deafness all have their onset near puberty and are more commonly associated with each other. None of these three responds well to penicillin treatment alone; often topical and or systemic corticosteroids are also necessary to halt progression. This triad therefore is considered by many to represent a type of hypersensitivity phenomenon rather than a purely spirochetal involvement of these structures. Recent evidence suggests that *T. pallidum* may persist for many years in the aqueous humor in cases of interstitial keratitis despite previous systemic therapy.

Serology in Pregnancy and the Newborn

Both reagin and treponemal antibodies as well as those antibodies responsible for a false positive reaction will cross

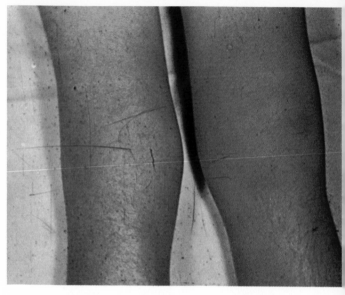

FIGURE 68. Congenital syphilis: Clutton's joints.

the placenta; therefore if the mother has a reactive serologic test for syphilis, one may expect the newborn's serologic test also to be reactive. The higher the titer of the mother's blood, the greater the chance that the newborn's serologic test will be reactive. If the mother has a high titer, the infant will probably have a high titer; however if this is due to passive transfer of antibody the child's titer should not exceed the mother's. A reactive serologic test in the newborn, due to passive transfer, should revert to nonreactive by 3-4 months of age; if it has not, active infection of the newborn is strongly suggested. A rising titer is diagnostic.

If the mother is infected late in the pregnancy, it is possible for both the mother and the newborn to have a nonreactive serologic test for syphilis at the time of delivery. In such a case, clinical signs and a rising titer in the ensuing weeks will confirm the diagnosis. As mentioned previously, treponemal antibodies also cross the placenta. Reactive TPI tests due to passive transfer of antibody have been reported in up to 100 percent of the newborns of TPI reactive mothers. (See "Serologic Interpretation," page 103).

Pregnancy itself is probably a very rare cause of false positive reaction. However, a false positive reaction due to other causes as are seen in the general population may also be seen in the pregnant female. Elevated reagin levels due to causes other than syphilis (false positive) in the pregnant female will also cross the placenta to produce a reactive serologic test for syphilis of a false positive nature in the newborn. This titer will also usually revert to nonreactive by 3 months of life. An acquired false positive in the infant is very rare before one-half year of life.

Bibliography

1. BROWN, WILLIAM J., AND MOORE, M. BRITTAIN: Congenital syphilis in the United States. Clin. Pediatrics, 2:220, May 1963.
2. CURTIS, ARTHUR C., AND PHILPOTT, JR., OSGOODE S.: Prenatal syphilis. M. Clin. North America, 48:707-719, May 1964.
3. KING, AMBROSE, AND NICOL, CLAUDE: Venereal Diseases. Philadelphia, F. A. Davis Co., 1964.
4. KONSTANT, GEORGE: Serology of syphilis in the newborn and infant. Dermat. Digest, 3:57, June 1964.
5. NABARRO, DAVID: Congenital Syphilis. London, Edward Arnold Ltd., 1954.
6. SARTAIN, PEGGY: The anemia of congenital syphilis. South. M.J., 58:27, January 1965.
7. THOMAS, EVAN W.: Syphilis: Its Cause and Management. New York, Macmillan Co., 1949.

Chapter IX.—SEROLOGIC INTERPRETATION

Human infection with *Treponema pallidum* stimulates the host's defense mechanisms and provokes a complex antibody response. The detection of one or another of these antibodies is the basis of serologic testing. The ideal single test would be easily and quickly performed, it would be highly sensitive and specific, and the results would be readily reproducible in different laboratories. At present, no such ideal test is available. Although over 200 tests for syphilis have been described, only a few are now used. By carefully selecting and familiarizing himself with two or three tests, the clinician may diagnose syphilis in nearly any stage using tests currently available.

No other tests employing immunologic methods have had such widespread use. Consequently, the standardization and performance of the tests are of utmost importance to insure uniform interpretation. The **sensitivity** of a test refers to its ability to be reactive in the presence of syphilis, while the **specificity** of a test refers to its ability to be nonreactive in the absence of the disease. Some highly sensitive tests are particularly suited for screening purposes; other tests are highly specific and assist in making problem diagnoses. Serologic tests are a definite aid in the diagnosis of syphilis in any stage, and they are the basis for the diagnosis of latent syphilis.

Classification of Tests

All tests for syphilis depend on the reaction of antibody with antigen. The tests may be classified by the type of antigen used. Nontreponemal or reagin tests are performed with extracts from normal tissue or other sources. Treponemal tests employ treponemes or treponemal extracts to detect antibody.

The reaction of antibody with antigen may be detected by various laboratory methods; the indicator system used allows a further classification of the treponemal and nontreponemal tests (Table 3). For example, the antibody (reagin) that reacts with purified beef heart extract (cardiolipin-lecithin) binds complement and prevents hemolysis of sensitized erythrocytes (the indicator system). The test is

TABLE 3. — Partial Classification of Tests for Syphilis

I. NONTREPONEMAL ANTIGEN TESTS

    Flocculation
        Venereal Disease Research Laboratory (VDRL) Slide
        Kahn Standard
        Kline
        Mazzini

    Complement Fixation
        Kolmer

    Agglutination
        Rapid Plasma Reagin

II. TREPONEMAL ANTIGEN TESTS

    Complement Fixation
        Reiter Protein Complement Fixation
        Kolmer with Reiter Protein Antigen
        Treponema pallidum Complement Fixation
        Treponema pallidum Cryolysis Protein

    Agglutination
        Treponema pallidum Agglutination

    Immobilization
        Treponema pallidum Immobilization (TPI)

    Immunofluorescence
        Fluorescent Treponemal Antibody (FTA–200)
        Fluorescent Treponemal Antibody Absorption
        (FTA–ABS)

nontreponemal; the reaction is demonstrated by complement fixation. An example of a nontreponemal complement fixation test is the Kolmer.

When antibody reacts with treponemes dried and fixed on a microscopic slide, the reaction may be demonstrated by the reaction of antisera to human immune globulin conjugated with a fluorescent dye. The Fluorescent Treponemal Antibody Absorption (FTA-ABS) test is a treponemal immunofluorescent test.

Nontreponemal Antigen Tests

Unless specifically noted to the contrary, use of the terms "serology," "serologic test," or "serologic reaction" in this book refers to nontreponemal antigen tests. Although these nontreponemal antigen tests are not absolutely specific or sensitive for syphilis, their performance is quite practical, they are widely available, and their findings are, without doubt, indicative of possible infection.

The original Wassermann test was a complement fixation test presumed to detect antibodies to treponemes. An extract of the liver of a syphilitic stillborn was used as antigen. It was later found, however, that normal liver extract served equally well in the test. The test that eventually developed was therefore a nontreponemal complement fixation test. Although the name "Wassermann" is still used by some to refer to any nontreponemal or serologic test for syphilis, the Wassermann test as such is no longer performed. For the sake of correct usage the term should be dropped.

Reactive nontreponemal tests confirm the diagnosis in the presence of early or late lesion syphilis; offer a diagnostic clue in latent, subclinical syphilis; are an effective tool for detecting cases in epidemiologic investigations; and are superior to the treponemal tests for following the response to therapy. The likelihood of obtaining a reactive VDRL or Kolmer test in untreated syphilis is shown in Table 4.

Reagin is first detected in the serum at approximately 4 to 6 weeks after infection, or 1 to 3 weeks after the chancre appears.

TABLE 4. — Comparative Sensitivity of Nontreponemal and Treponemal Tests in Untreated Syphilis

STAGE	APPROXIMATE PERCENT OF SERUMS EXPECTED TO GIVE REACTIVE TEST RESULTS				
	NONTREPONEMAL TESTS		TREPONEMAL TESTS		
	VDRL SLIDE	KOLMER	FTA–200	TPI	FTA–ABS
Primary	76	65	40	53	86
Secondary	100	100	95	98	100
Early Latent	95	95	90	94	99
Late Latent	72	65	68	89	96
Late (Tertiary) ..	70	60	77	93	97

Serial quantitative serologic examinations may reveal a dynamic process. A rising titer may indicate a recent infection, reinfection in an adequately treated patient, relapse in an inadequately treated patient, or an acute false positive reaction. Adequate treatment of early syphilis is shown by a decline in titer. Typical serologic responses following treatment are shown in Table 5. The number and frequency of quantitative serologic tests needed after treatment are given in the chapter on "Treatment," page 112. Titers should become nonreactive in 6 to 12 months following treatment for primary syphilis and in 12 to 18 months after treatment for secondary syphilis. Treatment of a late latent or late infection usually has little or no effect on the titer and should not be used to gauge the adequacy of treatment. Titers tend to become lower with time, but frequently remain reactive in low titer. The posttreatment titer in early latent syphilis may follow either the course of secondary or late latent syphilis. If the titer rises persistently (by at least two tube dilutions) it must be concluded that the disease remains active and retreatment must be initiated. A one tube variation up or down in quantitative titer is not considered significant because it is within the limits of

TABLE 5.—Typical Serologic Response to Therapy in Syphilis

Stage	Days after Therapy	Qualitative Methods		Quantitative Method VDRL Slide
		VDRL Slide	Kolmer[1]	
I. Primary Syphilis.	0	R	R 4+	R 2 dils
	32	R	4+	2 dils
	62	R	4+	2 dils
	96	WR	R 2+	WR 0 dils
	118	N	N	N
	165	N	N	N
	239	N	N	N
II. Secondary Syphilis.	0	R	R 4+	64 dils
	34	R	4+	32 dils
	65	R	4+	16 dils
	91	R	4+	4 dils
	118	R	R 3+	4 dils
	180	WR	R 1+	WR 0 dils
	245	N	N	N
	299	N	N	N
	348	N	N	N
III. Early Latent Syphilis.	0	R	R 4+	32 dils
	2	R	4+	16 dils
	36	R	4+	16 dils
	66	R	4+	8 dils
	100	R	4+	4 dils
	147	R	4+	8 dils

laboratory error (see examples III and IV, Table 5).

Careful attention must be paid to **every** reactive or weakly reactive serologic result. Many cases of untreated late latent or late syphilis will give only weakly reactive results with undiluted serum. On the other hand, the titer is usually high (16 dils or greater) in secondary syphilis. A high titer does not necessarily mean early syphilis (or even

TABLE 5.—Continued

STAGE	DAYS AFTER THERAPY	QUALITATIVE METHODS		QUANTITATIVE METHOD
		VDRL SLIDE	KOLMER[1]	VDRL SLIDE
	203	R	R 3+	2 dils
	266	WR	3+	WR 0 dils
	349	N	R 1+	N
	428	N	N	N
	510	N	N	N
IV. Late Latent Syphilis.	0	R	R 4+	8 dils
	9	R	4+	8 dils
	94	R	4+	4 dils
	178	R	4+	4 dils
	255	R	4+	8 dils
	360	R	4+	4 dils
	537	R	4+	2 dils
	709	R	4+	4 dils
	888	R	R 3+	2 dils
	1,061	WR	3+	WR 0 dils
	1,366	WR	3+	WR 0 dils
	1,651	WR	3+	WR 0 dils

SYMBOLS: N = nonreactive; WR = weakly reactive; R = reactive; dils. = abbr. for dilutions—the reciprocal of the highest titer giving a fully reactive test.

[1]In qualitative tests, numbers refer to the intensity (1–4) of the reaction in undiluted serum.

syphilis) but it is strong evidence for the presence of syphilis. Some of the highest titers recorded have been in late visceral or cutaneous syphilis or in nonsyphilitic diseases; e.g., hemolytic anemia or systemic lupus erythematosus.

Certain special purpose tests have been developed for rapid screening of sera. One of these is the Rapid Plasma Reagin (RPR) test. A modified VDRL antigen is used and the test is made more sensitive by the addition of choline chloride. Blood is collected in anticoagulant tubes, centrifuged, and tested immediately without heating the plasma.

The "RPR antigen" has been adapted to perform a similar test on the plasma portion of a microchematocrit determination (Plasmacrit or PCT test). After reading the packed cell volume, the capillary tube is divided and the plasma is expressed for testing. The PCT test has been especially useful in blood bank operation to exclude donors before collection, in screening hospital admissions, and, since capillary specimens are used, in testing infants. The Unheated Serum Reagin test (USR), another rapid screening test, is a further modification of the RPR test.

Reporting of Nontreponemal Antigen Tests

The result of qualitative tests for syphilis are customarily reported as **reactive** (or positive, or 4+), **weakly reactive** (or weakly positive, or 3+, 2+, or 1+), or **nonreactive** (negative.) Quantitative results may be obtained by diluting the serum in geometrical progression to an end-point. The titer is usually expressed as the highest dilution in which the test is fully reactive. In examples (a) and (b) below, the specimen was fully reactive at a dilution of 1 to 32 (1:32); this may also be expressed as "32 dils." Example (c) would be reported as reactive at 4 dils; example (d) weakly reactive, 0 dils.

The excessive production of antibody (particularly in the secondary stage of syphilis) occasionally results in the prozone phenomena due to the antibody excess. This is true of complement fixation or flocculation tests. Undiluted specimens will give a nonreactive or weakly reactive test result. Testing at higher dilutions, however, gives reactive test results. Example (e) is a prozonal reaction and would be reported as R 128 dils.

Serum Dilution

EXAMPLE	0	2	4	8	16	32	64	128	256
a)	4+	4+	4+	4+	4+	4+	2+	0	0
b)	R	R	R	R	R	R	WR	N	N
c)	R	R	R	WR	N	N			
d)	WR	N	N						
e)	N	WR	R	R	R	R	R	R	N

A few laboratories still report Kahn or Kolmer tests by multiplying the last reactive dilution by 4 and calling the product "Kahn units" or "Kolmer units" or simply "KU."

Treponemal Antigen Tests

Since the nontreponemal antigen tests are not entirely specific for *T. pallidum* infection, antigens for testing have also been prepared from treponemes. Some of the first tests developed with treponemal antigens are tedious to perform, expensive, and lack the sensitivity of nontreponemal tests. Treponemal tests are primarily used as confirmatory tests in diagnostic problem cases; e.g., patients in whom the clinical, historical, or epidemiologic evidence of syphilis is equivocal.

The *Treponema pallidum* Immobilization (TPI) test, while time consuming, technically difficult, and very expensive to perform, has been the standard by which all treponemal antigen tests are judged. This test employs as antigen living, virulent *T. pallidum* (Nichols strain) obtained from testicular syphilomas of infected rabbits. When syphilitic

103

serum and complement are added and incubated, the treponemes are immobilized; that is, they stop moving. The TPI becomes reactive later in early syphilis than the nontreponemal antigen tests since the TPI antibody develops more slowly. Therefore, some patients with primary syphilis who are reactive in the nontreponemal tests may have a nonreactive TPI test.

The Reiter Protein Complement Fixation test (RPCF) or Kolmer Test with Reiter Protein Antigen (KRP) utilized as antigen a protein fraction extract from the Reiter treponeme, a nonpathogenic cultivatable organism, and had the advantage of lower cost and ease of performance. When performed with proper controls according to published techniques, these tests were thought to give highly specific results. However, these tests have not lived up to their early promise with respect to specificity, and their greatest drawback is lack of sensitivity in syphilis of long duration.

The Fluorescent Treponemal Antibody (FTA) tests are the most recent and most promising tests to date. Antigen consisting of dead *T. pallidum* (Nichols strain) is allowed to dry on a slide and is overlaid with the unknown serum. Should the serum contain antibodies to *T. pallidum,* the antibodies will adhere and cover the organism with an invisible layer of antibody. This is then treated with fluorescein-tagged antibody to human globulin. If the globulin (syphilitic antibody) coats the treponeme, the tagged material reacts with it and the treponeme will fluoresce when viewed under ultra-violet light. No fluorescence is observed if syphilitic antibody is absent.

When the description of the FTA was first published a 1:5 dilution of serum in saline was employed and the test demonstrated good sensitivity and specificity. However, the sensitivity was greatly increased following the use of an improved fluorescein compound (fluorescein isothiocyanate) in the preparation of the specific conjugate. With th increase in sensitivity, nonspecific reactions were found to occur in approximately one-fourth of the general population. Quantitative studies indicated that these nonspecific reactions could be eliminated, for the most part, by testing a 1:200 dilution of the patient's serum. This modification of the FTA is called the FTA-200 and while it is less tedious and less expensive than the TPI, it is also less sensitive (Table 4). If serum is diluted 1:5 with an extract of non-pathogenic treponemes (Reiter), "group" treponemal antibodies are absorbed and "specific" antibodies remain in the syphilitic serum. This is the basis of the newest FTA test, the Fluorescent Treponemal Antibody Absorption (FTA-ABS) test. This test has been shown to be more sensitive than and at least as specific as any treponemal or non-treponemal test. The FTA-ABS test becomes reactive earlier than the TPI in early syphilis and it is about 5 percent more sensitive than the TPI in late latent or late syphilis (Table 4). The FTA-ABS test is now widely available and because of its increased sensitivity and specificity is the confirmatory test of choice.

False-Positive Reactors

Soon after the introduction of serologic tests for syphilis by Wassermann in 1906, Landsteiner and others suspected that some serums gave false-positive responses. This was later verified when tests detecting treponemal antibodies became available, since treponemal tests are capable of distinguishing latent syphilis from false-positive reactions. If one of the less sensitive treponemal tests is reactive, syphilis may be diagnosed. Should this test be nonreactive, the diagnosis of syphilis may not be excluded until a nonreactive TPI or preferably FTA-ABS is obtained.

All normal sera may contain minute amounts of reagin. The sensitivity of nontreponemal tests is altered by varying the proportion of reagents, temperature, mixing time, and other physiochemical variables. For these reasons, about one-fourth of all false-positive reactions represent technical errors or day-to-day variability in testing. Such titers rarely exceed weakly reactive or reactive at 1 dil. These "technical" false-positive reactors may be excluded by repeating the same nontreponemal tests and obtaining nonreactive results.

Repeatedly reactive nontreponemal tests accompanied by nonreactive treponemal tests (TPI or the more sensitive FTA-ABS) characterize the false-positive reactor. The duration of reagin reactivity arbitrarily determines whether the false-positive reaction is acute (less than 6 months) or chronic (6 months or longer). Though false-positive reactions have been called "biologic," many such reactions are associated with specific diseases or follow vaccination or immunization; therefore, this adjective is best discarded. To be descriptive, the terms acute false-positive or chronic false-positive adequately describe what is observed.

Acute false-positive reactions are found in persons suffering from many viral and bacterial infections or who have had certain vaccinations and immunizations. Titers are generally less than 8 dils; the reaction lasts a few weeks to a few months. Often, no pre-existing illness or specific cause may be recognized. A word of caution must be emphasized. A history of a prior infection or immunization in a patient with a low-titered STS in no way confirms a false-positive reaction. Syphilis is still the single most common cause of a reactive test for syphilis. Unless tests promptly become nonreactive or a nonreactive treponemal test result is obtained, syphilis cannot be reliably excluded.

Chronic false-positive reactions are usually less frequent than "technical" false-positive or acute false-positive reactions. Of nearly 700 cases of chronic false-positive reactors recorded in several carefully assembled series in the literature, about 50 percent were found initially in persons under 30 years of age, 70 percent are women, and about 10 percent have been associated with systemic lupus erythematosus. Some other patients have findings suggestive of collagen disease; still others are associated with the "autoimmune" group of diseases.

Lepromatous leprosy, heroin addiction, and occasionally malaria are associated with chronic false-positive nontreponemal tests for syphilis. The nonvenereal treponematoses (yaws, pinta, bejel) characteristically give reactive nontreponemal tests as well as treponemal tests and are not serologically distinguishable.

One more warning may be in order. Should the patient have multisystem disease and a positive LE cell preparation, a reactive serologic test is often considered automatically to be false. Syphilis and systemic lupus erythematosus or syphilis and leprosy can and do coexist. Each case must be determined individually by clinical appraisal and appropriate serologic tests.

Passive reaginemia is the term applied to placental transfer of maternal reagin to an uninfected newborn (congenital false-positive reactor). Antibodies crossing the placenta are predominantly of the type reacting in complement fixation tests; flocculation tests will give much lower titers in the neonate than in the maternal serum. Children born to women treated for syphilis during pregnancy are not always cured *in utero* (depending on drug, dosage, and duration of treatment). All children giving reactive tests at birth must be followed with serial serologic tests. A falling titer represents catabolic loss of passively transferred reagin; rising titers indicate active infection requiring treatment. Immobilizing antibodies may also passively cross the placenta and detectable levels may persist up to 6 months, occasionally giving reactive results for a longer period than the reagin tests.

If there is doubt about interpretation of treponemal tests results, consultation should be obtained from a syphilologist or a physician experienced in venereal disease control.

Bibliography

1. BRADFORD, LYNDA L., BODILY, HOWARD L., KETTERER, WARREN A., PUFFER, JEAN, THOMAS, JUNE E., AND TUFFANELLI, DENNY L.: FTA-200, FTA-ABS, and TPI tests in serodiagnosis of syphilis. Public Health Rep., 80:797-804, September 1965.

2. DEACON, WILBUR E., LUCAS, JAMES B., AND PRICE, ELEANOR V.: Fluorescent treponemal antibody-absorption (FTA-ABS) test for syphilis. JAMA, 98:624-628, November 7, 1966.

3. HUNTER, E. F., DEACON, W. E., AND MEYER, P. E.: An Improved FTA Test For Syphilis: The absorption procedure (FTA-ABS). Pub. Health Reports, 79:410-412, 1964.

4. MOORE, M. BRITTAIN, JR., AND KNOX, JOHN M.: Sensitivity and specificity in syphilis serology: clinical implications. South. M.J., 58:963-968, August 1965.

5. NICHOLAS, LESLIE, AND BEERMAN, HERMAN: Present day serodiagnosis of syphilis. Am.J.M.Sc., 249:466-483, April 1965.

6. OLANSKY, SIDNEY, AND NORINS, LESLIE C.: Current serodiagnosis and treatment of syphilis. JAMA, 198:165-168, October 1966.

7. TUFFANELLI, DENNY L., WUEPPER, KIRK D., BRADFORD, L. L., AND WOOD, R. M.: Fluorescent treponemal antibody tests for syphilis, New England J. Med., 276:258-261, February 2, 1967.

8. SMITH, J. LAWTON, AND ISRAEL, C. W.: The presence of spirochetes in late seronegative syphilis. JAMA, 199:980, March 27, 1967.

Chapter X.—TREATMENT

Those who treated their first case of syphilis with bismuth compounds and arsenicals can best appreciate the strides made in the treatment of syphilis in the last quarter of a century.

Over 20 years ago, Dr. John Mahoney working in the Venereal Disease Research Laboratory reported to the world the first cures of syphilis with penicillin. Much has happened to the World but not to syphilis since that momentous discovery. The causal treponeme has not developed any measurable resistance to the product of Fleming's antibacterial fungus and penicillin remains the best and most effective treatment of syphilis.

If the physicians of the Renaissance who watched this disease sweep Europe were alive today they would be most skeptical if they were told that there is a drug that with one injection will cure the "great pox" in its early stages. Even Ehrlich with his magic bullet, arsphenamine or 606, would have been astounded at penicillin's lack of toxicity as compared to his chemotherapeutic agent and would have had to acknowledge penicillin's more potent spirocheticidal action.

Following Mahoney's work with penicillin, the broad spectrum antibiotics were also found effective in the treatment of syphilis. However, these oral preparations are not preferred to penicillin for the following reasons:

1. Less spirocheticidal action (some are only static in action).
2. Absorption is highly variable.
3. Patient cooperation is not always obtained.

4. Follow-up studies still leave some doubt as to efficacy of treatment, especially when minimal doses are used in pregnancy and in obese individuals.

Penicillin

Any of the following three preparations may be used satisfactorily in the treatment of any of the stages of syphilis (see following treatment schedules, and Table 6, "Summary of the Management of Syphilis," page 112):

1. Benzathine penicillin G.
2. Procaine penicillin G with 2 percent aluminum monostearate (PAM).
3. Aqueous procaine penicillin G.

These preparations must all be administered intramuscularly. The use of oral penicillin is not recommended.

Broad Spectrum Antibiotics

When patient sensitivity to penicillin precludes the use of this drug, then erythromycin, tetracycline, chlortetracycline, oxytetracyline, and demethylchlortetracycline are the best alternate choices. In early syphilis the recommended total dosage for demethylchlortetracycline is 20-30 grams; if another tetracycline or erythromycin is given the dosage should be 30-40 grams. Treatment should be given 4 times daily in equally divided doses and extended over a period of 10-15 days. If these alternate broad spectrum antibiotics are employed, close follow-up of the syphilitic patient is imperative for the reasons mentioned earlier. This is especially true in pregnant females. It is also imperative that a spinal fluid examination be done as part of follow-up after this type of therapy. In late syphilis, cardiovascular syphilis, or neurosyphilis the total dosage should be doubled if any of these broad spectrum antibiotics are used in treatment.

Primary and Secondary Syphilis

Rx: Benzathine penicillin G: 2.4 million units total (1.2 million units in each buttock) by intramuscular injection at one clinic session.

or: PAM: 4.8 million units total usually given 2.4 million units at first session, as above, and 1.2 million units in each of 2 subsequent injections 3 days apart.

or: Aqueous Procaine penicillin G: 4.8 million units as total given 600,000 units daily for 8 days.

Latent Syphilis

Rx: Benzathine penicillin G: 2.4 million units as in primary syphilis.

or: PAM: 4.8 million units as in primary syphilis.

or: Aqueous Procaine penicillin G: 4.8 million units as in primary syphilis.

NOTE: If no spinal fluid examination is done, treatment must encompass the possibility of asymptomatic neurosyphilis and treatment should be given according to the schedule below.

Congenital Syphilis

Under 2 years of age.

Rx: Benzathine penicillin G—50,000 u/kg of body weight at one clinic visit.

or: Aqueous procaine penicillin G—100,000 u/kg (or 50,000/lb) of body weight divided into daily dosage over 10-day period.

Over 2 years but under 70 lb.

Rx: Benzathine penicillin G—50,000 u/kg of body weight at one clinic visit.

or: Aqueous procaine penicillin G—100,000 u/kg of body weight divided into daily dosage over 10-day period. Total dosage not to exceed 3,000,000 units.

TABLE 6. — Summary of the Management of Syphilis

STAGE	TREATMENT	FOLLOW-UP POSTTREATMENT	
		SEROLOGY	DISCHARGE[1]
Primary and Secondary	2.4 million units benzathine penicillin G, half in each buttock, single session.	1st, 3rd, 6th, 12th months.	End of 1 year.
Latent, both Early and Late..	If no spinal fluid examination: Total: 6.0 million units benzathine penicillin G. Initial: 3.0 million units, then 1.5 million units at 7-day intervals x 2. If spinal fluid examination is non-reactive: Total: 2.4 million units in single dose.	As above, then every 6 months for second year.	End of 2 years.
Syphilis in Pregnancy[2]	As above depending on stage.	Monthly until de-livery, then as for appropriate stage.	End of 1-2 years, depending on stage.
Subsequent pregnancies. No change in titer[2]	No treatment indicated.	Initial visit and monthly until delivery.	

	50,000 units benzathine penicillin G/Kg body weight in a single dose.[4]	Same as primary or secondary.	End of 1 year.
Early Congenital (under 2 years)[3]			
Late Congenital (over 2 years)[3]: Under 12 years: weight 70 lb. or less[3]	Same as early congenital.	Plus every 6 months for 2 years.	End of 2 years.
12 yr. or older but weight more than 70 lb.	Same as comparable adult stage.	Same	End of 2 years.
Neurosyphilis	Total: 6.0-9.0 million units benzathine penicillin G. Initial: 3.0 million units, then 3.0 million units every 7 days x 1 or 2.	Every 3 months for 1st year.	End of 2 years.
Cardiovascular Syphilis		Every 6 months for 2nd year.	
Late Benign Syphilis			

[1] A spinal fluid examination is suggested at the time of discharge for all patients with other than primary or secondary syphilis as discharge patients should have either negative serologic tests for syphilis or fixed low titers. Neurosyphilis patients should have a spinal fluid examination at each follow-up visit.

[2] Retreatment is indicated if there is any doubt concerning adequacy of previous treatment.

[3] An appropriate medical specialist should be consulted regarding treatment of the complications of congenital syphilis.

[4] Aqueous procaine penicillin G (page 111) is probably the preferred form of penicillin in the treatment of very small infants, because of the local irritant effect occasionally observed with benzathine penicillin G.

NOTE: When penicillin is contraindicated use: Tetracycline or Erythromycin: 750 mg every 6 hours for 10-15 days. In pregnancy, erythromycin for a full 15 days is preferred. The infant should be followed clinically and serologically for 3-4 months following birth. Tetracycline has been reported to cause dental staining and deformity when used in pregnancy and young children.

12 years or older, and/or weight more than 70 lb. (Same as for comparable stages of acquired syphilis).

Late Syphilis

(includes Neurosyphilis, Cardiovascular Syphilis, and Late Benign Syphilis)

Rx: Benzathine penicillin G: 6.0-9.0 million units total, given 3.0 million units initially, then 3.0 million units every 7 days x 1 or 2.

or: PAM: 6.0-9.0 million units total, given 1.2 million units at 3-day intervals.

or: Aqueous procaine penicillin G: 6.0-9.0 million units total, given 600,000 units daily. Any benefit from more than 10 million units has not been demonstrated.

Syphilis in Pregnancy

Generally speaking the pregnant woman with syphilis should be managed in the same manner as anyone else. However, urgency of diagnosis and treatment is the keynote. If she is sensitive to penicillin, then erythromycin is probably the broad spectrum antibiotic of choice, since staining and defective teeth not infrequently occur in children whose mothers were treated with tetracycline when *in utero*. It is frequently questioned as to whether it is necessary to retreat a woman in subsequent pregnancies or one who gives a history of syphilis and satisfactory treatment. In the days of arsenical (or pre-penicillin) treatment many clinicians stated emphatically that "every woman with a history of syphilis must be treated during each pregnancy." Today **one adequate course** of penicillin treatment suffices during the life of any syphilitic patient unless reinfection or relapse occurs. This rule applies to the pregnant woman as well, regardless of the time of previous treatment. However, all pregnant women previously treated for syphilis should have regular physical examinations and serologic tests at monthly intervals throughout pregnancy. Finally, if there is any doubt regarding the diagnosis or the adequacy of previous treatment, the patient should be retreated with a dosage that is known to be adequate.

Former Treatment

The physician is frequently confronted with older patients who have low titered reactive serologic tests and some history of arsenical and bismuth therapy. Metal therapy, while dangerous and long term, was effective when carried to completion. However, few individuals ever completed therapy which lasted $1\frac{1}{2}$ years. If it can be established with reasonable certainty that the patient has received a total of 20 arsenical and 20 bismuth injections within one year this is considered as constituting minimal effective therapy and further treatment is not indicated. Since adequate therapy histories often cannot be obtained, the physician is justified in retreating these patients with fully adequate dosages of penicillin in the same manner as if they were newly discovered cases of late latent syphilis. No form of heavy metal therapy is indicated in the modern day management of syphilitic patients.

Fever therapy was once an important adjunct in the treatment of neurosyphilis. Penicillin is unquestionably superior and completely supersedes this form of therapy.

Some physicians, in other areas of the world, still advocate the use of bismuth prior to penicillin in the treatment of cardiovascular and other forms of late syphilis. It is believed, however, that there is no sound evidence to indicate that preliminary bismuth therapy reduces the incidence or severity of Herxheimer or other untoward reactions.

Preventive Treatment (Epidemiologic or Prophylactic)

While every effort, including a complete physical examination, should be made to arrive at a diagnosis before administering preventive treatment to someone known to have been exposed to infectious syphilis, it is a fallacy to wait for the disease to develop to the clinical or reactive serologic stage, meanwhile allowing reinfection of treated patients and the infection of additional persons. Adequate preventive treatment consists of 2.4 million units of benzathine penicillin G.

It is important to remember that in early syphilis local or generalized lesions may fail to occur or may be so slight as to escape notice, and such symptomless infection may be unsuspected until a reactive serology at some later time leads to the diagnosis of syphilis. Whenever undetected syphilis exists, it can be spread.

Syphilis is usually related to promiscuity and contacts frequently are promiscuous individuals. It is not reasonable to suppose that clinicians can curtail the sexual activity of these contacts while they are incubating and developing the disease during the follow-up period. Preventive treatment is given for the purpose of destroying all treponemes of a contact with incubating syphilis, thus aborting the disease in its prodromal stage and rendering the patient incapable of spreading it to others.

Bibliography

1. ALLISON, J. RICHARD, JR.: Epidemiological treatment of syphilis. J. South Carolina M.A., 6:239-241, August 1965.

2. MOORE, M. BRITTAIN, JR., PRICE, ELEANOR V., KNOX, JOHN M., AND ELGIN, LEE W.: Epidemiologic treatment of contacts to infectious syphilis. Pub. Health Rep., 78:966-970, November 1963.

3. OLANSKY, SIDNEY, AND GARSON, WARFIELD: The treatment of syphilis with antibiotics other than penicillin. Arch. Dermat. Syph., 77:648-650, 1958.

4. Summary of the treatment of syphilis. Appendix in M. Clin. North America, 48:811-814, May 1964.

Chapter XI.—SPECIAL PROBLEMS OF DIAGNOSIS AND MANAGEMENT

Relapse and Reinfection

Relapse refers to the persistence, progression or reappearance of clinical, serological or laboratory evidence of disease following treatment. In early syphilis the differentiation between relapse and reinfection may be difficult, but the extreme efficacy of modern antibiotic treatment, particularly penicillin, minimizes the possibility of relapse. In early syphilis lesions disappear and the serological reagin titer decreases rapidly and regularly following adequate treatment. Failure to do so suggests reinfection or inadequacy of treatment. Reinfection may often be difficult to prove, but it is indicated by a new primary lesion at a site different from the initial primary lesion, a serological pattern of a first infection, and a history of new exposure. Both relapse and reinfection require retreatment (the former with double the recommended schedule), and also demand renewed epidemiological investigation.

In late syphilis, reinfection is unlikely even following treatment; relapse, however, may be a problem. In neurosyphilis the cerebrospinal cell count and protein should return to near normal levels within one year of treatment. Unfavorable clinical response or laboratory findings indicate the need for retreatment.

As discussed in the section on "Serologic Interpretation" page 99, syphilis of long duration characteristically produces a fixed, low-titered serology. No amount of treatment will revert this to nonreactive.

Finally, in pregnancy when any doubt exists about the adequacy of previous treatment or the presence of active infection, a course of treatment should be given for the prevention of congenital syphilis.

Jarisch-Herxheimer Reaction

The Jarisch-Herxheimer reaction, known in the older literature as therapeutic shock, is believed to be caused by the rapid release of antigenic materials from lysed treponemes. It is noted after the first injection of any potent treponemicidal drug and attests to the efficacy of the medication. A local and general reaction may occur. The local reaction consists of an intensification of the lesions. In primary syphilis the chancre may become edematous with concomitant increase in the size of the satellite bubo. A faint secondary rash may become prominent. Systemically there is frequently a rise in temperature to 101°-102° F., and rarely the temperature may reach 104° F. These reactions usually occur within 12 hours after initiation of treatment. The duration is usually only a few hours and rarely more than 24 hours. Herxheimer reactions are most marked in stages where treponemes are abundant. This includes early syphilis and general paresis. The ambulant patient should be informed that he may experience a self-limited febrile period following therapy. Symptomatic antipyretic and analgesic treatment is useful in reducing any discomfort.

Usually the Herxheimer reaction is benign and indicates a favorable response to treatment. In late syphilis the reaction can be more serious. Some paretics may have convulsions or increasing agitation requiring restraints or sedatives, but this is not an indication for discontinung treatment. It was originally thought that a local flare in cases of syphilitic aortitis might cause coronary occlusion or precipitate heart failure. Most of these data were collected in the pre-penicillin era and were probably due to the toxic effects of the drugs employed. Modern authorities recommend full therapeutic doses of penicillin or other effective antibiotics. If cardiac decompensation is present, this should receive initial consideration.

Allergic Reactions

Allergy, more properly called hypersensitivity, indicates a state of specifically altered reactivity dependent upon an antigen-antibody reaction. As such it is a type of immunity although, paradoxically, many times detrimental rather than protective. Two types of hypersensitivity reactions are generally distinguished on the basis of reaction time following a challenging dose of antigen. One is the immediate (humoral), and the other is the delayed (cellular) reaction. While different in almost all respects, both require an initial inductive or sensitizing dose of antigen before a reaction can occur. General characteristics of the immediate hypersensitivity reaction are passive transfer by serum or plasma; induction by injection of soluble antigens; reactions within minutes or hours; a basic vascular pathophysiology including edema, hyperemia, and endothelial swelling; and a rather easily produced desensitization. On the other hand, the delayed type is transferred by cells only; is induced by particulate matter, infection, or killed microorganisms; occurs within hours or days after challenge; has a basic cellular pathology, largely invasion by mononuclear cells and lymphocytes; and resists desensitization efforts.

Either or both of these mechanisms may be functioning in drug-inducted hypersensitivities. Clinically, the immediate reactions may be manifested by urticaria, angioneurotic edema, generalized pruritus, or anaphylactic shock. The delayed reaction may frequently take the form of contact dermatitis, skin rashes, bullous eruptions, and exfoliative dermatitis.

Serum sickness, while actually a much delayed immediate hypersensitivity reaction, may result when the injected

119

antigen is retained long enough to function both as the sensitizing and the challenging antigen. Patients with serum sickness will have fever, arthralgias, urticarias, and maculopapular skin eruptions occurring some 7 to 12 days after injection of the drug.

With the exception of anaphylactic shock which is discussed below, allergic reactions are generally successfully treated by antihistamines in milder cases and by corticosteroids in those that are more severe.

Anaphylaxis

Anaphylaxis is an immediate type of hypersensitivity where the antibody is thought to be fixed to the surface of mast cells or basophils. On reacting with the antigen various pharmacologically active compounds, including histamine, serotonin, and probably other less well-known substances, are released from the carrier cell. These released substances subsequently react on certain "end-organ" tissues including smooth muscle, connective tissue, and blood vessels. A shocklike state known as "anaphylaxis" may develop, and can be life-threatening.

Prime offender among substances known to precipitate these reactions is penicillin. It should never be administered to anyone giving a history of past reaction. Also, with those patients giving histories of other allergies or atopy caution is urged in its use. All patients should be closely observed for at least 20 minutes following penicillin administration, because serious anaphylactic reactions and death may occur unless immediate emergency measures are taken. Patients developing shock may have such prodromal symptoms as vertigo, nausea, flushing, pruritus, dyspnea, or abdominal pain. Audible wheezing, hypotension and tachycardia may be present. Treatment with 0.5 cc of 1:1000 epinephrine intramuscularly into the previous injection site frequently aborts progression of the syndrome.

If bronchospasm or laryngeal edema are not immediately relieved, or if the reaction appears explosive at its onset, intravenous epinephrine should be slowly administered. Epinephrine is the mainstay of treatment. However, other medications, including aminophylline, and antihistamines, or a soluble corticosteroid administered intravenously, may be needed. A running intravenous setup with a large-bore needle facilitates treatment. If hypotension occurs, vasopressors can be added to the intravenous solution. Should the emergency warrant, a tracheostomy and closed-chest cardiac massage may be life-saving.

It should be emphasized that most anaphylaxis has an unfavorable outcome because of failure to observe need for or tardiness in initiation of treatment.

Skin Testing

Penicillin has one of the highest therapeutic indices known, but paradoxically is the single substance most often implicated in anaphylaxis. While the exact incidence of penicillin hypersensitivity is unknown, a minimum of 1 person in 20 can be expected to exhibit some type of adverse reaction either so mild as to escape attention or so serious as to result in shock and death. Such deaths are extremely rare, with incidence of not more than 1 in every 78,000 patients treated.

To predict these adverse reactions by objective and reliable criteria would be most desirable. One approach has been skin testing utilizing dilute solutions of penicillin. This has included both the scratch and the intradermal techniques. Test results subsequently showed the former to be too insensitive and that both techniques possessed the capability of precipitating anaphylactic shock.

While a number of skin tests for penicillin hypersensitivity have been devised, including one in 1962 using penicilloylpolylysine, these tests leave much to be desired and

121

further studies are indicated.

At present alternate therapy should be given to patients giving a past history of penicillin sensitivity.

Bibliography

1. ARBESMAN, CARL E.: Clinical anaphylaxis and serum sickness. In Immunological Diseases, edited by Max Samter. Boston, Little, Brown, and Co., 1965, page 654.

2. BENDIXEN, GUNNAR: Classification of hypersensitivity in relation to clinical disease. Ann. Int. Med., 64:668-686, 1966.

3. DEWECK, A. L., AND BLUM, G.: Recent clinical and immunological aspects of penicillin allergy. Internat. Arch. Allergy, 27:221-256, 1965.

4. LEVINE, B. B., AND FELLNER, M. J.: The nature of immune complexes initiating allergic wheal and flare reactions. J. Allergy, 36:342-352, 1965.

5. WILLCOX, RICHARD R.: A Textbook of Venereal Diseases and Treponematoses. Second Edition. Springfield, Ill., Charles C. Thomas, 1964.

6. WILLCOX, RICHARD R.: Influence of penicillin allergic reactions on venereal disease control programs. Brit. J. Vener. Dis., 40:200-209, September 1964.

INDEX

Hutchinson's triad, **5, 89, 91;** infection of fetus after 18th week of gestation, **86;** interstitial keratitis, **5, 89;** Kassowitz' law, **86;** latency in, **5;** pathology of, **34-37;** serology of newborn in, **93-95**

    false positive reaction in, **93-95**

    early (before age 2), **87, 88, 111, 112-113**

        signs and symptoms of, **87, 88**

            anemia, **88;** bone involvement (osteochondritis), **87, 88;** central nervous system findings, in, **88;** cutaneous lesions, **87;** hepatosplenomegaly, **88;** mucous membrane lesions, **87**

    late (beyond age 2), **88, 89, 91, 93, 111, 112, 113, 114**

        is not infectious, **89**

        latent, **88, 89**

        signs of, **89, 91, 93**

            bone involvement (sabre shin, saddle nose configuration, perforation of hard palate), **91;** cardiovascular lesions, **91;** Clutton's joints, **93;** cutaneous involvement (rhagades), **91;** eighth nerve deafness, **91;** Hutchinson's teeth, **89, 91;** interstitial keratitis, **89;** mulberry or Moon's molars, **91;** neurosyphilis, **91**

    treatment of, **111, 112, 113, 114**

Control of Syphilis:

    adequate treatment, **12;** by incarceration and quarantine of persons thought infected with, **12;** by public health control measures, such as, **iii, 12, 13, 14, 15, 16, 70, 71, 72, 115, 116**

    case prevention through spread control (epidemiology), **12, 14, 15, 70-72, 115, 116**

        contact tracing, **70-72;** patient interview, **70;** preventive (epidemiologic or prophylactic) treatment, **12, 15, 72, 115, 116**

Chamberlain-Kahn Act, **13;** cooperation of physicians, public health workers, and citizens, **14, 16;** Lanham Act, **14;** mass serologic testing, **15;** National Venereal Disease Control Act, **14;** rapid treatment centers, **15;** Surgeon General's Task Force on Syphilis Eradication, **15;** Venereal Disease Division, U.S. Public Health Service, **13;** World War II impetus, **15**

Cullerier, M., **4**

D

Darkfield method, **8, 42, 43, 44, 87**

Diagnosis of syphilis:

    from darkfield examination of early lesion specimens, **43, 44**

        by identifying morphology and motility of *Treponema pallidum*, **43, 44;** by interpreting negative darkfield findings, **44**

    from medical history of patient, **41, 42;** from physical

examination, **42;** need for high index of suspicion in, **41;** neurosyphilis by spinal fluid examination, **44**

Diday, P., **5**

E

Eighth nerve deafness, **5, 91**

Ehrlich, Paul, **9, 10, 11, 13, 109**

Epidemiology:

basic concepts of, **70, 117**

every infectious case is considered a potential epidemic, **70;** in relapse and reinfection, **117;** trained epidemiologists assist in bringing infected contacts to treatment, **70**

contact tracing, **12, 13, 14, 15, 71, 72, 115, 116**

to ensure examination and treatment of infected contacts, **71, 72;** to give prophylactic treatment to not infected sexual contacts, **12, 16,· 71, 72, 115, 116;** to prevent disease spread, **14, 15, 70, 71**

patient interviewing, **70, 71**

to elicit sexual contacts, syphilis suspects or associates, **70, 71;** to find the source contact, **71;** to inform patient about his disease, **71**

Epidemiologic treatment.

(*See* Preventive treatment.)

F

False positive reactors:

acute, **106;** chronic, **106**

associated with lepromatous

leprosy, heroin addiction, and malaria, **107**

elimination of "technical", erroneous, **106;** in pregnancy and the newborn (passive reaginemia), **93, 107;** treponemal tests distinguish latent syphilis from, **105**

Fever (heat) therapy for syphilis, **4, 11, 12, 115**

by electronic cabinet, **12;** by malarial treatment, **11, 12**

Fleming, Alexander, **12, 109**

Fluorescent Treponemal Antibody Absorption (FTA-ABS) test, **105**

Fluorescent Treponemal Antibody (FTA) test, **104-105**

Fournier, Jean Alfred, **5**

Fracastorius, Hieronymus, **3-4**

G

Gale, Thomas, **4**

Gengou, Octave, **9**

Gilino, Corradino, **3**

Gonorrhea:

and syphilis, **6;** differentiation between, **7**

Grunpeck, Joseph, **6**

H

Hata, Sahachiro, **10**

Heat (fever) therapy for syphilis, **4, 11, 12, 115**

by electronic cabinet, **12;** by malarial treatment, **11, 12**

History of syphilis, **1-16**

Hoffman, Erich, **8, 13**

Hunter, John, **6**

Hutchinson, Jonathan, **5**

Hutchinson's teeth, **5, 89**

Hutchinson's triad:

eighth nerve deafness, **5, 89,**

95; pregnancy and congenital syphilis, **93, 94, 95**; pregnant mothers, **93, 94, 95, 107**; the newborn (passive reaginemia), **93, 94, 95, 107**

Snuffles, **87**

Specificity, **96**

Spinal fluid examinations:
in latent syphilis, **74**; in neurosyphilis, **79, 80, 81**
çerebrospinal fluid responses following treatment, **81**; for cell count, **79**; for reactive Kolmer or VDRL spinal fluid tests, **79, 80**; for total protein, **79**

Spirochaeta pallida (see *Treponema pallidum*):
as causative organism of syphilis, **8**; discovery of, **8**
in brain of paretic, **8, 9**; in human aorta, **8**

Spirochete, **17**

Syphilis:
acquired, **4, 5**
by infants, **4, 5**; latency in, **5**
cause of, theories of:
bacteria, **8**; humors of body, lack of balance of, **8**; *Spirochaeta pallida* (*Treponema pallidum*), **8**; stars and planets, malignant alignment of, **8**; *Treponema pallidum* (*Spirochaeta pallida*), **8**
clinical diagnosis of (*see* Diagnosis of syphilis); congenital (*see* Congenital syphilis); late (*see* Late syphilis); latent (*see* Latent syphilis)
origin, theories of:
bacteria, **8**; Columbian the-

ory of, **1, 2, 4**; epidemics of, **1, 2, 3**; first mention of, **3**; humors of body, lack of balance of, **8**; of early names for, **3**; pre-Columbian theory of, **2**; stars and planets, malignant alignment of, **8**
pathology of (*see* Pathology of syphilis); primary (*see* Primary syphilis); secondary (*see* Secondary syphilis); serologic detection of (*see* Serologic detection of syphilis); serologic tests for (*see* serologic tests for syphilis); treatment of (*see* Treatment of syphilis)

T

Tabes dorsalis, **5, 31, 33, 76, 77, 79, 91**
associated with optic atrophy, **79**; Charcot's joints in, **77**; in late congenital syphilis, **91**

Taboparesis, **79**. (*See* Paresis, **77**; Tabes dorsalis, **77, 79**.)

Terry, Luther, **15**

Treatment of syphilis:
allergic reactions (hypersensitivity to penicillin, **119-120**
definition of, **119**; types, of, **119**
delayed, **119**; immediate, **119**; serum sickness, **119, 120**
anaphylaxis, **120, 121**
cause of, **120**; definition of, **120**; management of, **120, 121**; symptoms of, **120, 121**
congenital, **111, 112-113**; in pregnancy, **86, 112-113, 114, 115, 118**; in relapse and rein-

131

—78° C, **22;** rabbit as experimental host for, the, **22;** susceptibility to heat, drying, soap and water, and refrigerator temperature, **22**
Treponema pallidum Immobilization (TPI) test, **103, 104**
Treponema pertenue, **17**
Treponemataceae, the family, **17**
 genera of, the, **17**
  Borelia, **17;** *Treponema,* **17;** *Leptospira,* **17**
Trousseau, **4**

U

Uhlenhuth, **10**

Unheated Serum Reagin (USR) test, **102**

V

Vallambert, Simon de, **5**
Verneuil, Aristide August, **6**
Vigo, Juan de, **3**
Villalobos, Francisco Lopez de, **3**

W

Wagner-Jauregg, Julius von, **11**
Wallace, William, **7**
Wassermann, August von, **9, 13, 98, 105**
 test, **98**
Wegner, G., **5**
Widmann, Johannes, **3**